The Book of Acupuncture Points

Compiled By

Dr. James Tin Yau So

Volume One
of
A Complete Course in Acupuncture

Paradigm Publications Brookline, Massachusetts
1985

The Book of Acupuncture Points
Compiled By
Dr. James Tin Yau So

ISBN 0-912111-02-X

Library of Congress Cataloging in Publication Data

So, James Tin Yau, 1911—
A Complete Course in Acupuncture

Includes index
Contents: v. 1. The Book of Acupuncture Points.
1. Acupuncture——Collected works. I. Title.
{ DNLM: 1. Acupuncture. WB 369 S675c }
RM184.S65 615.8'92 84—9478
ISBN 0—912111—02—X

Published by:
Paradigm Publications
44 Linden Street
Brookline Massachusetts 02146

This book was produced and typeset using software and services provided by Textware International of Cambridge Massachusetts.

Cover design by Herb Rich III
Caligraphy by 朱春汉题 Chun-Han Zhu, O.M.D.

Preface

I first met Dr. James Tin Yau So in 1972. I was brought to his school by my first teacher, Dr. Gin Shek Ju, who said "This man is famous throughout the East for his knowledge and understanding of the essence of acupuncture, and what is more important, he is truly a teacher!" At that time Dr. So had been teaching acupuncture in Hong Kong continuously since 1941.

At his college in Hong Kong his lectures were clear, concise and always practical. His students came from all over the Orient to attend his lectures. In Hong Kong I was at first his student, but then more importantly we became friends. At his request I made arrangements for him to come to the United States. We lived together in Los Angeles and developed the UCLA Acupuncture Project. Dr. So was always teaching, always helping others to understand acupuncture. In 1974 we moved to Boston setting up clinics and research programs, but still always teaching. I was able to help him set up the first full scale training program in this country: "The James/Stevens Acupuncture Center." Always teaching, always explaining, Dr. James So is currently the Founder and Principal Instructor Emeritus of the New England School of Acupuncture.

In this volume, his first published text, Dr. So contributes a major work to our knowledge of acupuncture. This is a compilation of understanding and experience, the distillation of the wisdom of a practitioner and clinician. This book includes exact locations of points based on tradition, experience and research. For the first time many different and effective techniques of treatment are discussed and delineated. Important therapeutic approaches to many common problems are clearly presented.

This text represents a milestone in the field. It brings the tradition, wisdom and experience of the East and its most illustrious clinician to the inquiring young students and practitioners in the West. He is still teaching, still explaining. It is with a great deal of pride, love and respect that I preface this book by Dr. James Tin Yau So, a teacher and a friend, a man well deserving the title by which he is known, "The Father of American Acupuncture."

Steven L. Rosenblatt, PhD.
President
California Acupuncture College
August 7, 1983

Foreword

James Tin Yau So and this book, **The Points of Acupuncture**, serve as a bridge between two cultures. Dr. So is part of a lineage involving an oral tradition in acupuncture. His teachers include Tsang Tien Chi, a student of Chang Tan An. Dr. So first came to the U.S.A. in 1973. Dr. So has maintained a remarkable depth of commitment and discipline in bringing acupuncture to the West. He has served in many acupuncture clinics throughout Asia and the United States. As a U.S. citizen, he has bridged traditions by compiling records of oral teachings, traditional textual material and notes on clinical experience into a clear, concise, highly relevant, practice-oriented text for his students. Dr. So, until recently, continued to practice the art and science of acupuncture in teaching clinics. His accessibility, openness and honesty in dealing with any acupuncture-related question defy the stereotype image of the Oriental mystique.

Dr. So is an empiricist. He teaches only what he knows, from his clinical experience, to be useful for helping patients. After more than 30 years of personal observation and clinical trials with acupuncture, Dr. So has eliminated or modified clinical teaching materials found to be invalid. His close scrutiny of patient-related therapeutic processes has led to the selection of the particularly powerful acupuncture point combinations for individuals with specific health problems.

Dr. So does not try to explain why his methods work. As a matter of history, he has commented upon the theory of Five Phase Evolution, also known as Five Elements. He considers the theory useful for talking about acupuncture, but not as important for good therapeutic results. Rather, he gives more emphasis to precise point location and the specific effects of acupuncture stimulation at these points.

This text serves as a needed reference guide for the objectification of acupuncture therapies. Knowledge of point location and the indications and contraindications of treatment techniques is basic to the further validation of acupuncture. The development of acupuncture as a safe or clinically useful method depends upon international exchange of information. Standardization of the name and location of points, specifics of point reaction, rationale for point selection and therapeutic combinations are necessary steps for further development of acupuncture as a valid clinical tool in western medical settings. Variability in the teachings of point location and point reaction is to be expected, as oral traditions are metaphorically rich, but not always precise. As a physician, medical educator and a student of cultural health care systems, I believe this text should serve as a standard reference for acupuncture clinical trials in the United States.

R. Prasaad Steiner, M.D.
President, Transcultural Health
Louisville, Kentucky 40204-4594

Associate Professor
Department of Family Practice
University of Louisville Medical School
Louisville, Kentucky 40292

Introduction to the Series

by
Dr. James Tin Yau So, N.D.

In the early part of this century, before 1930, very few people practiced acupuncture in South China. Traditional herbal medicine and Western allopathic medicine were prevalent. In Canton, there was only one well-known acupuncturist, a Buddhist monk.

It was in these surroundings that my teacher, Tsan Tien Chi, decided to study acupuncture. Why did a high school teacher make this decision? To start, his mother died of dropsy; Western medicine and herbs were of no help. His oldest son contracted a disease and died after severe vomiting and diarrhea. His second son died of dysentery. Later his wife was hospitalized for five days and almost died.

Tsang Tien Chi himself had asthma and external piles for over ten years. Western medicine and surgery had no lasting effect on his condition. He resolved to find an effective treatment.

In 1930, a friend of Tsang's from Shanghai told him that acupuncture could cure him and that acupuncture could be learned well in a short period of time. Tsang quit his job, sold his property and went to Shanghai. There he studied acupuncture at the school of the famous master, Ching Tan An.

After only one year Tsang returned to South China. Under his direction his wife treated him for asthma and piles and he was cured. In a short time he had many patients.

Two years later in 1934, Tsang opened a school, The College of Scientific Acupuncture in Canton, China. It was at that school that I learned acupuncture. While still a student I treated over 200 patients. One of these was my father who had asthma. After only three acupuncture treatments he never had another attack of asthma.

In 1939 I graduated and opened an office in Hong Kong. In 1941 I opened my own school, the Hong Kong College of Chinese Acupuncture. As of 1972 I had graduated 500 students. In 1973 I came to the United States and practiced in Washington D.C. Later that same year, I was invited by the University of California, Los Angeles, to be the senior acupuncturist for a pain control research project.

In 1974 I started practicing with other acupuncturists at the China Acupuncture Center in Boston. 1975 was a busy year. My students Arnie Frieman and Steven Breecher, M.D. and I started a school. Another student and I finished the first translation of **The Complete Course of Chinese Acupuncture**.

Between 1975 and 1982 I taught over 400 students at the New England School of Acupuncture. These students have had great success with the treatments in these books. I hope the reader will utilize the contents herein and help many patients.

Autobiography

Many students have asked me about myself and the origin of my skills and this book. In these pages, I will explain a little about both.

When I was very young, my father brought me to Hong Kong and took me to the Christian Church. There, I accepted God.

My interest was so great that, at age 17, I taught a Sunday School Class. Our church had many evangelical meetings. I always attended these.

In 1929, I studied to be a Christian preacher. By the time I was twenty years old, I was invited to be a regular preacher in the Assembly of God Church. I worked for ten years in Mainland China.

God always blessed me in everything I did. God performed many miracles to help me, but this is another story. I always resisted temptation and kept my body holy.

When Japan invaded China, the church closed. At that time I learned acupuncture from Tsang Tien Chi. Shortly after, I opened my clinic.

While practicing acupuncture, I always charged my patients very little. My treatments were available to the poor as well as to the rich. My business grew as my patients referred other patients. This made the patients happy and me happy. God, step by step, guided me to come and work in America in 1973.

Later, when the acupuncture business was slow, I still enjoyed myself every day. There was no need to worry about the future as God would take care of me.

I thought of going back to Hong Kong, but a friend founded a school for me and, later, I obtained a permanent resident card. The school kept me in America.

By my nature, I like to make a joke. I always like to laugh, and hear people laugh and enjoy each other. A Chinese proverb explains that laughter keeps you young; anger makes you old. Now, I am over 73, but I look much younger. People have asked me, "What is your secret of staying young?" The answer is to enjoy yourself every day. This is a difficult lesson to learn.

- You must not be greedy.
  Be satisfied with whatever you have.

- You must not be jealous of others.

- You must not get angry at others.
  Don't hold on to your anger.

- Don't worry about the future;
  believe that God will take care of you.

- Do not make any enemies.

- Forgive everybody and love them.

If you do all this, you will be happy and relaxed all the time. Your body's internal organs will function well and you will not suffer with disease.

Why is there so much cancer? Because people are not happy. The unhappiness causes abnormal organ function and then diseases such as cancer or high blood pressure will appear.

If you enjoy life everyday, your body will stay young with no disease.

The important thing is to believe in God. Don't do anything wrong and God will keep you healthy and happy. This is what I did and I believe it.

I have written this book to improve the practice of acupuncture and help more people be healthy.

In China, acupuncture teachers will only share 80% of what they know. I teach all I know to my students. I'm getting old; I can't work any more, so I teach my students to help others. In this way, I am still able to help many people.

I always enjoyed helping my patients. Now I enjoy my students helping them. I am satisfied that what I taught is good for the students and good for the world.

In return, I get a lot of love from my students and my patients. This makes me very happy. I will enjoy this the rest of my life.

Dr. James Tin Yau So, N.D.
September 1, 1983

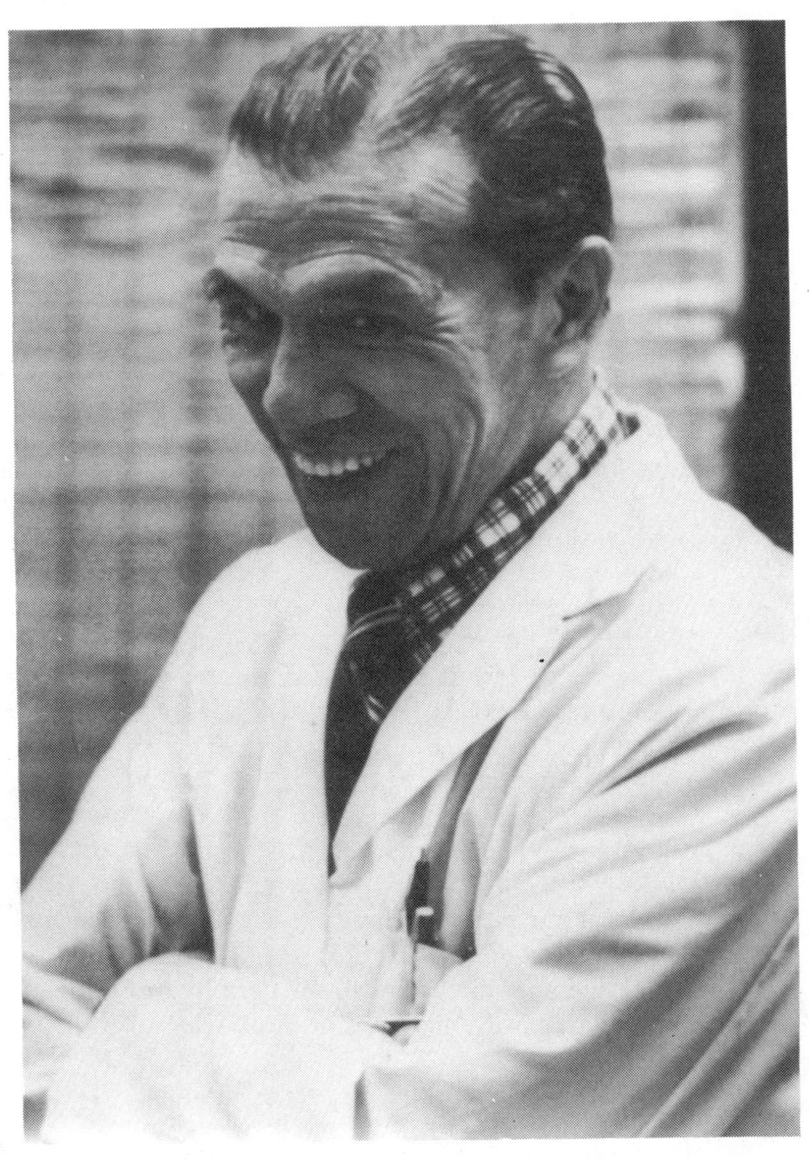

Dr. James Tin Yau So

Introduction

The Points of Acupuncture

There are many acupuncture books in the stores written by many different authors. Most of these books are translations or compilations from older Chinese books. This point book is different from the others in the following ways:

> The Mandarin names of the points in this book are spelled phonetically to make it easier for the English-speaking reader. I have tried to be as accurate, yet simple, as possible. Even so, there may be a few mistakes. Please note that this book does not use the type of Romanized spelling which is so popular in Asia but not in America.
>
> Following the descriptions in this book, the acupuncture points are easy to locate. These descriptions were developed by me during the course of 35 years of teaching acupuncture.
>
> You will not need a chart to locate the points.
>
> On most standard charts, 90 percent of the points are located correctly. The others are located incorrectly. This book includes directions in the description of the location to adapt any chart to this book.
>
> How do I know that this percentage of standard locations are incorrect? My teacher, Tsang Tien Chi, researched the points for many years. It is because of his work that I am sure the locations in this book are nearly 100 percent correct. If you do not believe this, I invite you to try these locations. You will believe these locations are correct; they work very well.

There are many points on the body which lie over a palpable pulse. Few, if any, other books describe which points these are and how to insert the needle without causing bleeding.

Included in every point description is the stimulus sensation which needs to be elicited for the point to be effective. There are very few books, if any, which have given the stimulus for every point.

If you locate the points correctly, the stimulus sensation will follow the prescribed path. This shows that your technique is correct.

The older books called the stimulus "Chi" and said, "You must elicit the Chi to get the desired effect." Chi is the power of the nerve. I have described the stimulus for over 400 points. Perhaps a few are incorrect. Also, on some people the nerve has grown in a slightly different direction, so the stimulus may follow a different path. Nonetheless, be sure to elicit some stimulus from the point.

Acknowledgements

I wish to thank Miss Karen Freede for taking one year of her life to help me translate the **Book of Acupuncture Points**, and the **Book of Acupuncture Technique**.

John V. Braga, who studied with me in Hong Kong over twenty five years ago, devoted himself tirelessly to translating **The Treatment of Disease by Acupuncture**. My sincerest appreciation goes to him.

I also wish to thank my student, Joseph S. Burstein, CA., for helping me to edit and arrange the present volumes and charts. Without his help these books would not be published.

Sincerely,

Dr. James Tin Yau So

About This Book

This, **A Complete Course in Acupuncture, Volume One**, is *Points of Acupuncture* in its entirety with the addition of comprehensive indexes. This book has had a number of preliminary editions and releases in English both as class notes and as a publication of the New England School of Acupuncture. This edition, the first complete edition assembled under the supervision of Dr. So himself, has been authorized, extensively checked, verified and extended. Many of his students have participated in the process of its assembly to insure that the oral tradition of Dr. So's teaching has been accurately reflected.

This volume is the first of two and covers the point locations, use of various needle and moxa techniques, contraindications and, uniquely, the stimulus to be expected from effective treatment of the point. The second volume covers the treatment of specific symptoms, diseases and cases according to the clinical experience of the author. Volume two includes the complete texts of **The Treatment of Disease by Acupuncture** and **The Book of Acupuncture Techniques.**

The editorial goal of the production has been to present as closely as is possible the knowledge of Dr. So's lifework as he wishes to present it. We have tried not to impose the mechanics and conventions of book publishing on what is largely an oral tradition and a personal style. We have sought to bring to print as directly as possible the experience of the author. Thus, the book has been designed as a text and reference work. The points discussed are divided into two sections. The first covers the most frequently used points by the anatomical area of their locations. The second section completes the point discussions meridian by meridian. In most cases a point description is complete within one page to make classroom and clinical use easy.

There are a number of point identifying systems in use, three basic transliteration systems, at least three meridian abbreviation schema and two styles of Chinese characters. Resolution of these various standards is left to others. The system used in this book utilizes capital letters for the meridian abbreviation and arabic numbers for the points. For each point there are three independant identifications: a meridian abbreviation and point number in series; a section number; and the Chinese name. The Chinese point names are represented by a phonetic spelling of the pronunciation of the Chinese characters, as well as an English translation. Both have been chosen by Dr. So and reflect his usage. Points are cross referenced by meridian, number and page. An index introduction has been provided for those who wish to use this feature. Computer database entries for each point are available.

For convenience of reference and to facilitate classroom use each of the body areas has been given a section number. Each point within that section is given a sequence number. Thus "5.12 " is the twelfth point of the fifth anatomical or meridian section. Illustrations of each of these body areas precede the discussions of the individual points and are referenced by the section number. The table of contents includes these identifiers so that reference should be consistent and simple even for beginning students who do not immediately associate a general location with a meridian name and point number.

For each point discussed, the **Location**, **Effects**, **Treatment** and **Stimulus** are given. **Location** is the means and measurements for locating the point. The descriptions are as much as possible "landmarks" which can be used regardless of the reader's facility with anatomical language. The divisions used as measurements are detailed separately. The **Effects** listed for each point include symptoms, disease names, and Chinese energetic concepts. The **Treatment** heading denotes both needle and moxa instructions. The **Stimulus** heading is a description of the patient's response to insertion at this point when the point is accurately located and properly treated.

The vocabulary of the **Effects** sections is as literal as possible a refection of the original Chinese meaning. Several of the expressions deserve note. "Melancholy" references an uncomfortable condition usually of the stomach and "sadness in the heart" is mental depression. "Overcooling" is a state of very low body temperature, pale face and lips, an empty condition. Its compliment, "overheating," is a full condition characterized by a very high temperature. "Confinement" is the traditional period of rest after childbirth. All references to the "old book" or "old books" are generalized references to the whole body of classical texts, not any particular text.

A few effects referenced require some familiarity with classical Chinese medical literature. These are present for practitioners who wish to take advantage of the research of Dr. So and his teachers. For example, Dr. So's indication that PC-7, Da Ling, is effective for a case of the "heart suspended as though hungry" seems enigmatic. However, it is a clear reference to the **Great Compendium**, Da Cheng:

> "Pain or malaise in the heart, feeling that the heart is hanging with a hungry feeling at the same time; pain in the heart with the palms of the hands very warm; pain in the chest and in the heart with moaning and anxiety."

Dr. So's clinical experience is extensive. He has practiced in circumstances where no other remedy was available. Often his practice has been the only medicine for large populations. Dr. So's references to advanced conditions, epidemics and terminal situations are literal and it should not be assumed that these treatments have been supplemented with other therapies.

Table of Contents

Measurement

Subject	Illus.	Page
Measurement of the Body		1
Division Measurement		1
Arm and Leg Division Measure	1	1
Measurement of the Head		2
Eye Division	2	2
Head and Face Lateral Measurements		2
Upper Chest Measurement		2
Trunk Lateral Measurements		2
Abdomen Measurement		2
Spine Measurement		3
Back Lateral Measurement		3
Front of Body Division Measure	3	4
Back of Body Division Measure	4	5
Acupuncture Meridians		6
Making Division Measurements		7
Division Measurement Chart		8

Points on the Head

Point	Pronunciation	Translation	Section	Illus.	Page
GV-24	Shen Ting	*spirit courtyard*	1,1	5	11
GV-23	Shang Hsing	*upper star*	1,2	5	11
GV-22	Shin Hui	*meeting of the skull bones*	1,3	5	12
GV-21	Chien Ding	*anterior summit*	1,4	5	12
GV-20	Bai Hui	*hundred meetings*	1,5	5	13
GV-19	Hou Ding	*posterior summit*	1,6	5	13

Top of Head, Bilateral

Point	Pronunciation	Translation	Section	Illus.	Page
GB-15	Lin Chi	*temporary crying*	2,1	5	14
GB-16	Mu Chuang	*eye window*	2,2	5	14

Points Around the Temples

Point	Pronunciation	Translation	Section	Illus.	Page
GB-13	Ben Shen	*natural spirit*	3,1	6	16
ST-8	Tou Wee	*head binding*	3,2	6	16

Back of Head and Neck

Point	Pronunciation	Translation	Section	Illus.	Page
GV-16	Feng Fu	*wind mansion*	4,1	6	17
GV-15	Ya Men	*door of muteness*	4,2	6	18
BL-10	Tin Chu	*pillar of heaven*	4,3	6	18
GB-20	Feng Chi	*wind pond*	4,4	6	19

Area Around The Ear

Point	Pronunciation	Translation	Section	Illus.	Page
TW-21	Er Men	*ear door*	5,1	7	21
GB-2	Ting Hui	*meeting of hearing*	5,2	7	21
SI-19	Ting Gung	*palace of listening*	5,3	7	22
TW-17	Yi Fung	*wind block*	5,4	7	22
ST-6	Jia Che	*chariot of the jaw*	5,5	7	23

Area Around the Eyes

Point	Pronunciation	Translation	Section	Illus.	Page
GB-14	Yang Bai	*yang white*	6,1	8	25
BL-2	Ts'uan Jhu	*drilling bamboo*	6,2	8	25
TW-23	Si-Jhu Kung	*silk bamboo hollow*	6,3	8	26
BL-1	Jing Ming	*eye bright*	6,4	8	26
GB-1	Tung-Tzi Liao	*bone hole of eye*	6,5	8	27

Points Around the Nose

Point	Pronunciation	Translation	Section	Illus.	Page
GV-25	Su Liao	*pure white bone hole*	7,1	9	29
LI-20	Ying Hsiang	*accept fragrance*	7,2	9	29

Points Around the Mouth

Point	Pronunciation	Translation	Section	Illus.	Page
GV-26	Shui Kou,	*water ditch,*			
	Ren Jung	*middle of man*	8,1	10	31
ST-4	Ti T'sang	*earth granary*	8,2	10	31
CV-24	Cheng Jiang	*receiving starch*	8,3	10	32

Special Points on the Head and Neck

Point	Pronunciation	Translation	Section	Illus.	Page
XN-1	Pak Loh	*one hundred labors*	9,1	11	34
XH-1	Er Jen	*upper point of ear*	9,2	11	34

XH-2	Sen Chung	*God's cleverness*	9,3	11	35
XH-3	Dang Yang	*during the yang*	9,4	11	35
XH-4	Faht Jei	*hair line*	9,5	11	36
XF-1	San Cha	*trigeminal*	9,6	11	36
XF-2	Tai Yang	*solar*	9,7	11	37
XF-3	Yin Tang	*hall of seal*	9,8	11	37
XF-4	Yu Yao	*fish loins*	9,9	11	38
XF-5	Pie Yen	*eyes of the nose*	9,10	11	38
XF-6	Jia-Cheng Jiang	*beside receiving starch*	9,11	11	38
XF-7	Hai Chuen	*sea spring*	9,12	11	39
XF-8	Jin Jin (left)	*golden fluid*	9,13	11	39
XF-8	Yu-Yeh (right)	*jade fluid*	9,14	11	39

Neck and Chest Area

Point	Pronunciation	Translation	Section	Illus.	Page
CV-23	Lien Ch'uan	*pure spring*	10,1	12	41
CV-22	T'ien T'u	*heavenly rushing*	10,2	12	42
CV-17	Shin Jung Tang Jung	*in the middle of the fat*	10,3	12	43
CV-16	Jung Ting	*middle courtyard*	10,4	12	43

Chest and Flank Area

Point	Pronunciation	Translation	Section	Illus.	Page
ST-12	Ch'ueh Pen	*broken basin*	11,1	13	45
ST-16	Ying Chuang	*chest window*	11,2	13	45
ST-18	Ru Gun	*root of breast*	11,3	13	46
LV-14	Chi Men	*waiting door*	11,4	13	46
LU-1	Chung Fu	*middle mansion*	11,5	13	47
LV-13	Jang Men	*seal door*	11,6	13	48
GB-26	Dai Mo	*waistband pulse*	11,7	13	49

Upper Abdomen, Center Line

Point	Pronunciation	Translation	Section	Illus.	Page
CV-15	Chiu Wei	*turtledove tail*	12,1	14	51
CV-14	Jiuh Chueh	*great palace gate*	12,2	14	52
CV-13	Shang Goan	*upper stomach*	12,3	14	52
CV-12	Jung Goan	*middle stomach*	12,4	14	53
CV-11	Chien Li	*established mile*	12,5	14	53
CV-10	Shia Goan	*lower stomach*	12,6	14	54
CV-9	Shui Fen	*divided water*	12,7	14	54
CV-8	Shen Chueh	*God's palace gate*	12,8	14	55

Lower Abdomen, Center Line

Point	Pronunciation	Translation	Section	Illus.	Page
CV-7	Yin Jiao	*yin transfer*	13,1	15	57
CV-6	Chi Hai	*sea of chi*	13,2	15	58
CV-5	Shi Men	*stone door*	13,3	15	59
CV-4	Kuan Yuan	*gate origin*	13,4	15	60
CV-3	Jung Ji	*middle extremity*	13,5	15	61
CV-2	Chu Gu	*crooked bone*	13,6	15	62
CV-1	Hui Yin	*perineum*	13,7	15	62
XSC-1	Nang Di	*bottom of scrotum*	13,8	15	63
XP-1	Gwie Tau	*head of penis*	13,9	15	64

Lower Abdomen, Lateral Two Divisions

Point	Pronunciation	Translation	Section	Illus.	Page
ST-25	Tien Shu	*heavenly pivot*	14,1	16	66
ST-27	Da Jiuh	*big great*	14,2	16	67
ST-28	Shui Dao	*water path*	14,3	16	67
ST-29	Gui Lai	*coming back*	14,4	16	68
ST-30	Chi Chung	*chi rushing*	14,5	16	68
LV-11	Yin Lian	*screen of sexual organ*	14,6	16	69

Points in the Shoulder Area

Point	Pronunciation	Translation	Section	Illus.	Page
GB-21	Jian Jing	*shoulder well*	15,1	17	71
LI-15	Jian Yu	*shoulder bone*	15,2	17	72
LI-16	Jiuh Guu	*great bone*	15,3	17	72

Midline of the Back, Governing Vessel

Point	Pronunciation	Translation	Section	Illus.	Page
GV-14	Da Chui	*big hammer*	16,1	18	74
GV-13	Tao Dao	*pottery path*	16,2	18	75
GV-12	Shen Juh	*body pillar*	16,3	18	76
GV-11	Shen Dao	*spirit path*	16,4	18	76
GV-10	Ling Tai	*spirit tower*	16,5	18	77
GV-9	Jyh Yang	*extreme yang*	16,6	18	77
GV-4	Ming Men	*gate of life*	16,7	18	78
GV-3	Yang Guan	*gate of yang*	16,8	18	79
GV-2	Yao Yu	*loins yu*	16,9	18	79
GV-1	Chang Chyang	*long strong*	16,10	18	80

Points Lateral One and One Half Divisions from Spine

Point	Pronunciation	Translation	Section	Illus.	Page
BL-11	Da Chu	*big shuttle*	17,1	19	82
BL-12	Feng Men	*wind gate*	17,2	19	83
BL-13	Fei Yu	*lung yu*	17,3	19	83
BL-15	Shin Yu	*heart yu*	17,4	19	84
BL-17	Ger Yu	*diaphragm yu*	17,5	19	84
BL-18	Gan Yu	*liver yu*	17,6	19	85
BL-19	Dan Yu	*gallbladder yu*	17,7	19	85
BL-20	Pe Yu	*spleen yu*	17,8	19	86
BL-21	Wei Yu	*stomach yu*	17,9	19	86
BL-22	San Jiao Yu	*triple warmer yu*	17,10	19	87
BL-23	Shen Yu	*kidney yu*	17,11	19	88
BL-25	Da Chang Yu	*large intestine yu*	17,12	19	89
BL-27	Shiao Chang Yu	*small intestine yu*	17,13	19	89
BL-28	Pang Guang Yu	*bladder yu*	17,14	19	90
BL-30	Bai Huan Yu	*white circle yu*	17,15	19	90
BL-31	Shang Liao	*upper sacral foramen*	17,16	19	91
BL-32	Tsie Liao	*second sacral foramen*	17,17	19	91
BL-33	Jung Liao	*middle sacral foramen*	17,18	19	92
BL-34	Hsia Liao	*lower sacral foramen*	17,19	19	92
BL-35	Hui Yang	*meeting of the yang*	17,20	19	93

Lateral Three Divisions From Spine

Point	Pronunciation	Translation	Section	Illus.	Page
BL-38	Gao Huang Yu	*area between the pericardium and heart*	18,1	20	95
XB-1	Pee Gun	*root of tumor*	18,2	20	96
BL-47	Tzee Shih	*palace of semen*	18,3	20	97
XB-2	Yao Yen	*eye of lumbar*	18,4	20	97

Points on the Arms and Hands

Point	Pronunciation	Translation	Section	Illus.	Page
LU-5	Chih Tzer	*foot marsh*	19,1	21	99
LU-7	Lieh Ch'ueh	*broken line*	19,2	21	100
LU-8	Jing Chyu	*meridian gutter*	19,3	21	101
LU-9	Tai Yuan	*bigger abyss*	19,4	21	101
LU-11	Shao Shang	*young merchant*	19,5	21	102
PC-3	Chu Tzer	*crooked marsh*	19,6	21	103
PC-4	Hsih Men	*door of the wall hole*	19,7	21	103

XA-1	Erh Bai	*double white*	19,8	21	104
PC-5	Jian Shih	*intermediary messenger*	19,9	21	104
PC-6	Ney Guan	*inner gate*	19,10	21	105
PC-7	Da Ling	*big mound*	19,11	21	105
PC-8	Lao Gung	*labor palace*	19,12	21	106
PC-9	Jung Chung	*middle rushing*	19,13	21	107
HT-3	Shaw Hai	*young sea*	19,14	21	108
HT-4	Ling Dao	*soul path*	19,15	21	109
HT-5	Tung Lie	*through a mile*	19,16	21	109
HT-6	Yin Hsi	*wallhole of the yin*	19,17	21	110
HT-7	Shen Men	*spirit door*	19,18	21	111
HT-8	Shaw Fu	*yang mansion*	19,19	21	112
HT-9	Shaw Chung	*lesser rushing*	19,20	21	113
XFi-1	Sze Fung	*four sewing*	19,21	21	113

Large Intestine Meridian

Point	Pronunciation	Translation	Section	Illus.	Page
LI-1	Shang Yang	*merchant yang*	20,1	22	115
LI-4	Ho Ku	*union of the valleys*	20,2	22	115
LI-5	Yang Hsi	*yang stream*	20,3	22	116
LI-10	(Shou) San Li	*arm three miles*	20,4	22	117
LI-11	Chu Chih	*crooked pond*	20,5	22	118
LI-13	Wu Li	*five miles*	20,6	22	119
LI-14	Bei Nau	*forearm*	20,7	22	119

Triple Warmer Meridian

Point	Pronunciation	Translation	Section	Illus.	Page
TW-1	Kuan Chung	*gate rushing*	21,1	23	121
TW-2	Yih Men	*fluid door*	21,2	23	121
TW-3	Jung Juu	*middle islet*	21,3	23	122
TW-4	Yang Chih	*yang pond*	21,4	23	122
TW-5	Wai Guan	*outer door*	21,5	23	123
TW-6	Chih Kou	*branch ditch*	21,6	23	123

Small Intestine Meridian

Point	Pronunciation	Translation	Section	Illus.	Page
SI-1	Shao Tzer	*young marsh*	22,1	24	125
SI-3	Hou Hsi	*back stream*	22,2	24	125
SI-4	Wan Gu	*wrist bone*	22,3	24	126
SI-5	Yang Guu	*yang valley*	22,4	24	126

SI-8	Hsiao Hai	*small sea*	22,5	24	127
XA-2	Jhou Jian	*sharp point of elbow*	22,6	24	127
XFi-2	Jung Kuei	*middle leader*	22,7	24	128
XFi-3	Dah Shiao Guu Kung	*big and small hollows*	22,8	24	128
XHn-1	Bah Hsieh	*eight ghosts*	22,9	24	129
XFi-4	Sih Shuian	*ten drain off*	22,10	24	129
XFi-5	Wu Fu	*five tigers*	22,11	24	130
XFi-6	Wen Tao	*tip of crease*	22,12	24	130

Spleen Meridian

Point	Pronunciation	Translation	Section	Illus.	Page
SP-1	Yin Bai	*hidden white*	23,1	25	132
SP-2	Dah Du	*big capital*	23,2	25	132
SP-4	Gung Sun	*grandfather grandson*	23,3	25	133
SP-5	Shang Chiu	*merchant hill*	23,4	25	133
SP-6	San Yin Jiao	*three yin crossing*	23,5	25	134
SP-9	Yin Ling Chuan	*yin hill stream*	23,6	25	135
SP-10	Sheue Hai	*sea of blood*	23,7	25	135

Liver Meridian

Point	Pronunciation	Translation	Section	Illus.	Page
LV-1	Da Duen	*big heap*	24,1	26	137
LV-2	Shing Jian	*walk in between*	24,2	26	137
LV-3	Tai Chung	*bigger rushing*	24,3	26	138
LV-4	Jung Feng	*middle seal*	24,4	26	138
LV-7	Shi Guan	*knee gate*	24,5	26	139
LV-8	Chu Chuan	*crooked spring*	24,6	26	139

Kidney Meridian

Point	Pronunciation	Translation	Section	Illus.	Page
KI-1	Yung Chuan	*bubbling up spring*	25,1	27	141
KI-2	Ran Gu	*blazing valley*	25,2	27	142
KI-3	Tai Hsi	*bigger stream*	25,3	27	143
KI-6	Jiu Hai	*shining sea*	25,4	27	144
KI-4	Da Jung	*big bell*	25,5	27	145
KI-7	Fu Liu	*returning current*	25,6	27	145
KI-8	Jao Shin	*exchanging letters*	25,7	27	146

Stomach Meridian

Point	Pronunciation	Translation	Section	Illus.	Page
ST-33	Yin Shih	*yin market*	26,1	28	148
XL-1	Shi Yan	*eyes of the knee*	26,2	28	148
XL-1a	Shi Yik	*wings of the knee*	26,3	28	149
XL-2	Hok Deng	*top of the crane*	26,4	28	149
ST-36	Tsu San Li	*leg three miles*	26,5	28	150
ST-36a	Lan Wei	*appendix*	26,6	28	150
ST-40	Feng Lung	*abundant bulge*	26,7	28	151
ST-41	Shye Shi	*loosening stream*	26,8	28	151
ST-42	Chung Yang	*rushing yang*	26,9	28	152
ST-44	Nei Ting	*inner courtyard*	26,10	28	152
ST-45	Li Dui	*sharpening exchange*	26,11	28	153
XT-1	Tu Yin	*single yin*	26,12	28	153

Bladder Meridian

Point	Pronunciation	Translation	Section	Illus.	Page
BL-50	Cheng Fu	*receive and accept*	27,1	29	155
BL-54	Wei Jung	*entrusting middle*	27,2	29	155
BL-57	Cheng Shan	*supporting mountain*	27,3	29	157
XL-3	Shan Sha	*below the mountain*	27,4	29	157
BL-60	Kuen Lun	*Kuen Lun mountain*	27,5	29	158
BL-62	Shen Mo	*extended meridian*	27,6	29	158
BL-63	Jin Men	*golden gate*	27,7	29	159
BL-67	Jih Yin	*extremity of yin*	27,8	29	159

Gall Bladder Meridian

Point	Pronunciation	Translation	Section	Illus.	Page
GB-30	Huan Tiao	*jumping circle*	28,1	30	161
XL-4	Huan Jung	*middle of the circle*	28,2	30	161
GB-31	Feng Shi	*wind market*	28,3	30	162
GB-33	Yang Guan	*knee yang gate*	28,4	30	162
GB-34	Yang Ling Chuan	*yang hill spring*	28,5	30	163
GB-38	Yang Fu	*yang support*	28,6	30	163
GB-39	Shuan Jung Jueh Gu	*suspended bell*	28,7	30	164
GB-40	Chiu Shu	*hill market*	28,8	30	164
GB-44	Chiao Yin	*foot hole of the yin*	28,9	30	165
XFo-1	Ba Feng	*eight winds*	28,10	30	165
XSP-1	Wah Toh Jet Jih	*Wah Toh's extra spleen point*	28,11	30	166

Conception Vessel Meridian

Point	Pronunciation	Translation	Section	Illus.	Page
CV-18	Yu Tang	*jade hall*	29,1		169
CV-19	Zi Gung	*purple palace*	29,2		169
CV-20	Hua Gai	*splendid covering*	29,3		170
CV-21	Xuan Ji	*pearl and jade*	29,4		170

Governing Vessel Meridian

Point	Pronunciation	Translation	Section	Illus.	Page
GV-5	Shuan Shu	*suspended pivot*	30,1		171
GV-6	Ji Jung	*middle of spine*	30,2		171
GV-7	Jung Shu	*middle pivot*	30,3		171
GV-8	Gin Shu	*contracted nerve*	30,4		172
GV-17	Nau Hoo	*brain door*	30,5		172
GV-18	Chiang Jian	*strength in between*	30,6		172
GV-27	Dui Duan	*extreme exchange*	30,7		173
GV-28	Y'n Jiao	*gum crossing*	30,8		173

Lung Meridian

Point	Pronunciation	Translation	Section	Illus.	Page
LU-2	Yun Men	*cloud door*	31,1		174
LU-3	Tian Fu	*heavenly mansion*	31,2		174
LU-4	Xia Bai	*chivalry white*	31,3		175
LU-6	Kung Tsui	*supreme hole*	31,4		175
LU-10	Yu Ji	*fish border*	31,5		176

Heart Meridian

Point	Pronunciation	Translation	Section	Illus.	Page
HT-1	Ji Chuan	*extreme spring*	32,1		177
HT-2	Ching Ling	*green spirit*	32,2		177

Pericardium Meridian

Point	Pronunciation	Translation	Section	Illus.	Page
PC-1	Tian Chi	*heavenly pond*	33,1		178
PC-2	Tian Chuan	*heavenly spring*	33,2		178

Large Intestine Meridian

Point	Pronunciation	Translation	Section	Illus.	Page
LI-2	Erh Jien	*second interval*	34,1		179
LI-3	San Jian	*third interval*	34,2		179
LI-6	Pian Lih	*inclined passage*	34,3		180
LI-7	Wen Liu	*warm current*	34,4		180
LI-8	Xia Lian	*lower screen*	34,5		181
LI-9	Shang Lian	*upper screen*	34,6		181
LI-12	Joou Liao	*elbow bone*	34,7		182
LI-17	Tian Ding	*heavenly vessel*	34,8		183
LI-18	Fu Tu	*support and rush*	34,9		183
LI-19	Ho Liao	*grain bone*	34,10		184

Triple Warmer Meridian

Point	Pronunciation	Translation	Section	Illus.	Page
TW-7	Hui Jung	*meeting ancestor*	35,1		185
TW-8	San Yang Lo	*3 yang binders*	35,2		185
TW-9	Si Du	*four gutters*	35,3		185
TW-10	Tian Jing	*heavenly well*	35,4		186
TW-11	Ching Leng Yuan	*pure cold abyss*	35,5		186
TW-12	Hsiao Leh	*thawing Leh River*	35,6		187
TW-13	Nao Hui	*arm meeting*	35,7		187
TW-14	Jian Liao	*shoulder bone*	35,8		187
TW-15	Tian Liao	*heavenly bone*	35,9		188
TW-16	Tin Yau	*window of heaven*	35,10		188
TW-18	Chi Mo	*madness pulse*	35,11		189
TW-19	Lu Xi	*skull rest*	35,12		189
TW-20	Jiao Sin	*angle of the ear*	35,13		190
TW-22	Ho Liao	*harmony bone*	35,14		190

Small Intestine Meridian

Point	Pronunciation	Translation	Section	Illus.	Page
SI-2	Chien Ku	*front valley*	36,1		191
SI-6	Yang Lao	*supporting the old*	36,2		191
SI-7	Jie Jeng	*support straight*	36,3		192
SI-9	Jian Jieng	*shoulder chastity*	36,4		192
SI-10	Nau Yu	*shoulder blade yu*	36,5		192
SI-11	Tien Jung	*heavenly ancestor*	36,6		193
SI-12	Bin Feng	*facing the wind*	36,7		193

SI-13	Chu Yuan	*crooked wall*	36,8		193
SI-14	Jian Wai Yu	*outside of the shoulder yu*	36,9		194
SI-15	Jian Jung Yu	*middle of the shoulder yu*	36,10		194
SI-16	Tian Chang	*heavenly window*	36,11		194
SI-17	Tien Yung	*heavenly appearance*	36,12		195
SI-18	Chuan Liao	*cheekbone hole*	36,13		195

Kidney Meridian

Point	Pronunciation	Translation	Section	Illus.	Page
KI-5	Shui Chuan	*water spring*	37,1		196
KI-9	Chu Bin	*building guests*	37,2		196
KI-10	Yin Gu	*yin valley*	37,3		197
KI-11	Heng Gu	*transverse bone (pubis)*	37,4		197
KI-12	Da Heh	*big brightness*	37,5		198
KI-13	Chi Hsueh	*chi hole*	37,6		198
KI-14	Szi Men	*four full*	37,7		198
KI-15	Jung Ju	*middle injection*	37,8		199
KI-16	Fong Yu	*vital yu*	37,9		199
KI-17	Shang Chu	*merchant's tune*	37,10		199
KI-18	Shi Guan	*stone gate*	37,11		200
KI-19	Yin Du	*ghost's capital*	37,12		200
KI-20	Tung Gu	*penetrating valley, abdomen*	37,13		200
KI-21	You Men	*gate of hades*	37,14		201
KI-22	Bu Long	*walking corridor*	37,15		201
KI-23	Shen Feng	*spirit seal*	37,16		201
KI-24	Ling Shu	*spirit market*	37,17		202
KI-25	Shen Tsang	*spirit store*	37,18		202
KI-26	Yu Jung	*amidst elegance*	37,19		202
KI-27	Yu Fu	*yu mansion*	37,20		203

Spleen Meridian

Point	Pronunciation	Translation	Section	Illus.	Page
SP-3	Tai Bai	*supreme whiteness*	38,1		204
SP-7	Lou Gu	*leaky valley*	38,2		204
SP-8	De Jee	*earth secret*	38,3		205
SP-11	Jee Men	*basket door*	38,4		205
SP-12	Chung Men	*rushing door*	38,5		206
SP-13	Fu Sheh	*mansion cottage*	38,6		206

Point	Pronunciation	Translation	Section	Illus.	Page
SP-14	Fu Jie	*abdomen knot*	38,7		207
SP-15	Da Heng	*big horizontal*	38,8		207
SP-16	Fu Ai	*abdomen sorrow*	38,9		208
SP-17	Shi Dou	*food drain*	38,10		208
SP-18	Tian Xi	*heavenly stream*	38,11		209
SP-19	Shung Shiang	*chest village*	38,12		209
SP-20	Jou Yung	*encircling glory*	38,13		210
SP-21	Da Bao	*big enveloping*	38,14		210

Liver Meridian

Point	Pronunciation	Translation	Section	Illus.	Page
LV-5	Li Kou	*insect ditch*	39,1		211
LV-6	Jung Du	*middle capital*	39,2		211
LV-9	Yin Bao	*yin wrapping*	39,3		212
LV-10	Wu Li	*(foot) 5 mile*	39,4		212
LV-12	Ji Mai	*quick pulse*	39,5		212

Stomach Meridian

Point	Pronunciation	Translation	Section	Illus.	Page
ST-1	Cheng Chi	*receive tears*	40,1		213
ST-2	Si Bai	*four whites*	40,2		213
ST-3	Ju Liao	*great bone*	40,3		214
ST-5	Da Ying	*big welcome*	40,4		214
ST-7	Shia Guan	*lower gate*	40,5		215
ST-9	Yen Ying	*man welcome*	40,6		215
ST-10	Shui Tu	*water rushing*	40,7		216
ST-11	Chi She	*chi shelter*	40,8		216
ST-13	Chi Hu	*chi cottage*	40,9		216
ST-14	Fu Fong	*treasure house*	40,10		217
ST-15	Wu Yi	*room screen*	40,11		217
ST-19	Bu Yung	*no admittance*	40,12		217
ST-20	Cheng Man	*receiving fullness*	40,13		218
ST-21	Liang Men	*beam door*	40,14		218
ST-22	Guan Men	*gate door*	40,15		218
ST-23	Tai Yii	*bigger one*	40,16		219
ST-24	Hua Rou Men	*slippery meat door*	40,17		219
ST-26	Wai Ling	*outside hill*	40,18		219
ST-31	Bi Guan	*thigh gate*	40,19		220
ST-32	Fu Tu	*crouch rabbit*	40,20		220
ST-34	Liang Chiu	*beam hill*	40,21		220
ST-35	Du Bi	*calf nose*	40,22		221

ST-37	Shang Ju Su	*upper great void*	40,23		221
ST-38	Tiao Kou	*line mouth*	40,24		222
ST-39	Sia Ju Su	*lower great void*	40,25		222
ST-43	Shian Gu	*sinking valley*	40,26		223

Gall Bladder Meridian

Point	Pronunciation	Translation	Section	Illus.	Page
GB-3	Shang Guan	*upper gate*	41,1		224
GB-4	Han Yan	*jaw detested*	41,2		224
GB-5	Shuan Lu	*suspended skull*	41,3		225
GB-6	Shuan Li	*suspended balance*	41,4		225
GB-7	Chu Bin	*twisted hair*	41,5		226
GB-8	Shuai Gu	*leading valley*	41,6		226
GB-9	Tien Chung	*heavenly rushing*	41,7		226
GB-10	Fu Bai	*floating white*	41,8		227
GB-11	Chiao Yin	*the yin of a hole*	41,9		227
GB-12	Wan Ku	*final bone*	41,10		228
GB-17	Cheng Ying	*upright camp*	41,11		228
GB-18	Cheng Ling	*receiving spirit*	41,12		228
GB-19	Nao Kong	*brain hollow*	41,13		229
GB-22	Yuan Yeh	*liquid of deep waters*	41,14		229
GB-23	Che Jin	*flank muscle*	41,15		230
GB-24	Yih Yueh	*sun and moon*	41,16		230
GB-25	Jing Men	*capital door*	41,17		231
GB-27	Wu Shu	*five pivots*	41,18		231
GB-28	Wei Dao	*blinding path*	41,19		232
GB-29	Ju Liao	*dwelling bone*	41,20		232
GB-32	Jung Du	*middle ditch*	41,21		232
GB-35	Yang Jiao	*yang crossing*	41,22		233
GB-36	Wai Chiu	*outer mound*	41,23		233
GB-37	Guang Ming	*light bright*	41,24		234
GB-41	Lin Chi	*(foot) above tears*	41,25		234
GB-42	Di Wu Hui	*earth five meetings*	41,26		235
GB-43	Shia Shi	*chivalrous stream*	41,27		235

Bladder Meridian

Point	Pronunciation	Translation	Section	Illus.	Page
BL-3	Mei Chung	*eyebrow raising*	42,1		236
BL-4	Chu Cha	*crooked officer*	42,2		236
BL-5	Wu Chu	*five places*	42,3		236
BL-6	Cheng Kuang	*receive light*	42,4		237

BL-7	Tung Tien	*penetrate heaven*	42,5	237
BL-8	Lo Chueh	*connecting deficient*	42,6	238
BL-9	Yu Jeen	*jade pillow*	42,7	238
BL-14	Chuh Yin Yu	*absolute yin yu*	42,8	238
BL-16	Du Yu	*governing vessel yu*	42,9	239
BL-24	Chi Hai Yu	*sea of chi yu*	42,10	239
BL-26	Guan Yuan Yu	*gate origin yu*	42,11	239
BL-29	Jung Lu Yu	*middle of the backbone yu*	42,12	240
BL-36	Fu Fen	*supplementary division*	42,13	240
BL-37	Po Hu	*strength house*	42,14	241
BL-39	Shen Tang	*spirit hall*	42,15	241
BL-40	Yi Shi	*sighing giggling*	42,16	241
BL-41	Ge Guan	*diaphragm gate*	42,17	242
BL-42	Hwen Men	*soul door*	42,18	242
BL-43	Yang Gang	*yang bound*	42,19	242
BL-44	Yi Sheh	*thought shelter*	42,20	243
BL-45	Wei Tsang	*stomach granary*	42,21	243
BL-46	Huang Men	*vitals door*	42,22	243
BL-48	Bao Huang	*womb and vitals*	42,23	244
BL-49	Jih Bian	*folding edge*	42,24	244
BL-51	Yi Men	*prosperous gate*	42,25	244
BL-52	Fu Shi	*floating accumulation*	42,26	245
BL-53	Wei Yang	*commanding yang*	42,27	245
BL-55	Ho Yang	*uniting yang*	42,28	245
BL-56	Cheng Jin	*supporting nerves*	42,29	246
BL-58	Fei Yang	*flying high*	42,30	246
BL-59	Fu Yang	*foot bone yang*	42,31	247
BL-61	Pu Tsan	*official's aide*	42,32	247
BL-64	Jing Gu	*capital bone*	42,33	248
BL-65	Shu Gu	*bind the bone*	42,34	249
BL-66	Tung Gu	*penetrating the valley*	42,35	249

Measurement of the Body

I. Division Measurement

For use in measuring along the length of the patient's arms and legs, measure the distance between the dorsal edge of the two distal creases of the bent middle finger of patient's left hand (if female, measure the right hand). This is one division.

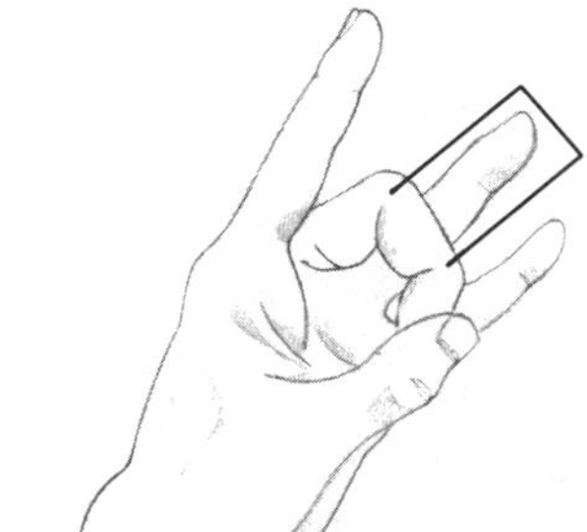

Arm and Leg Division Measure
Illustration 1

From wrist crease to elbow crease, along the inside of the arm, is twelve divisions. From elbow crease to the tip of the shoulder joint is twelve divisions. From the tip of the prominence of the femur at the hip to the crease behind the knee is eighteen divisions. From the crease behind the knee to the external prominence of the ankle bone is sixteen divisions.

II. Measurement of the Head

Head divisions do not correspond to arm or leg divisions.

From the front hairline to the back hairline is twelve divisions. However, for a balding patient, the distance is measured from between the two eyebrows to the back hairline and is fifteen divisions. This means that the forehead is three divisions. From the front hairline to the C7↔T1 intervertebral space is fifteen divisions. From the back hairline to C7↔T1 intervertebral space is three divisions. If the back hairline is irregular, use the measurement from the front hairline to the hollow at the base of the skull. This is eleven divisions.

III. Head and Face Lateral Measurements

For use in laterally measuring the head and face, measure the width of the patient's eye from the inner corner to the outer corner, along the bottom of the eyelid, while the eye is open.

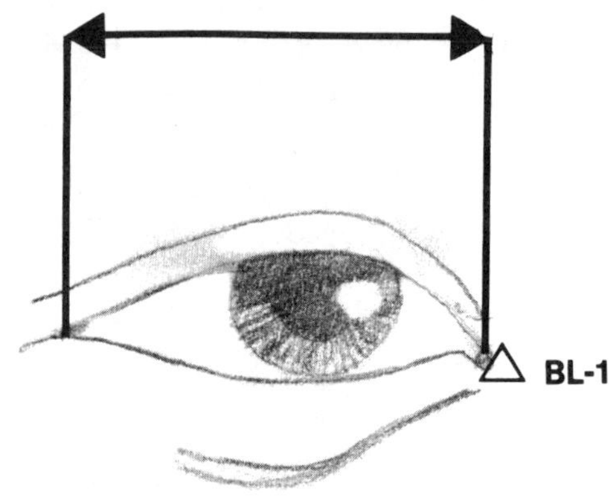

Eye Division
Illustration 2

IV. Upper Chest Measurement

By custom, each rib is 1 and 3/5 divisions apart.

V. Trunk Lateral Measurements

The distance between the center of the patient's nipples is eight divisions.

VI. Abdomen Measurement

From the bottom of the xyphoid process to the middle of the umbilicus is eight divisions. All body charts showing seven divisions are wrong. If there is no xyphoid process, find the hollow at the lower edge of the sternum. The distance between this hollow and the middle of the umbilicus is nine divisions. From the middle of the umbilicus to the upper edge of the pubic bone is five divisions.

VII. Spine Measurement

The spine is measured by counting each intervertebral space, and is divided into five sections:

Section	Vertebra
Cervical vertebrae	7
Thoracic vertebrae	12
Lumbar vertebrae	5
Sacral vertebrae	5, partly fused
Coccyx	divided into 4 segments

VIII. Back Lateral Measurement

Lateral measurement of the back uses the division based on a patient's middle finger.

Division Measures
Front of Body

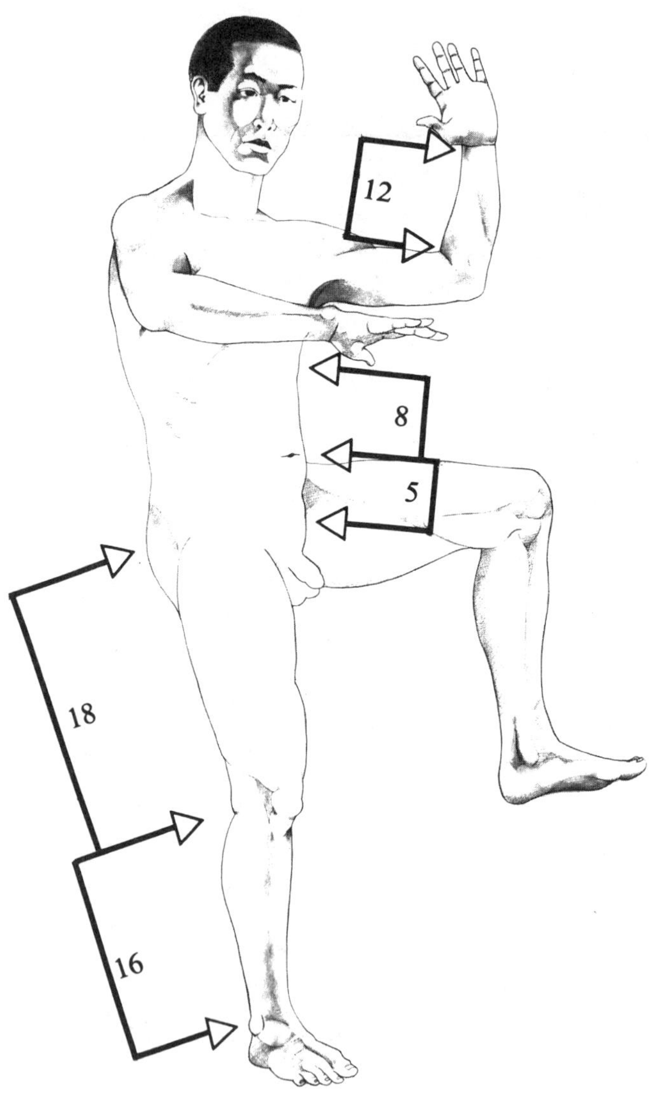

Front of Body Division Measure
Illustration 3

Division Measures
Back of Body

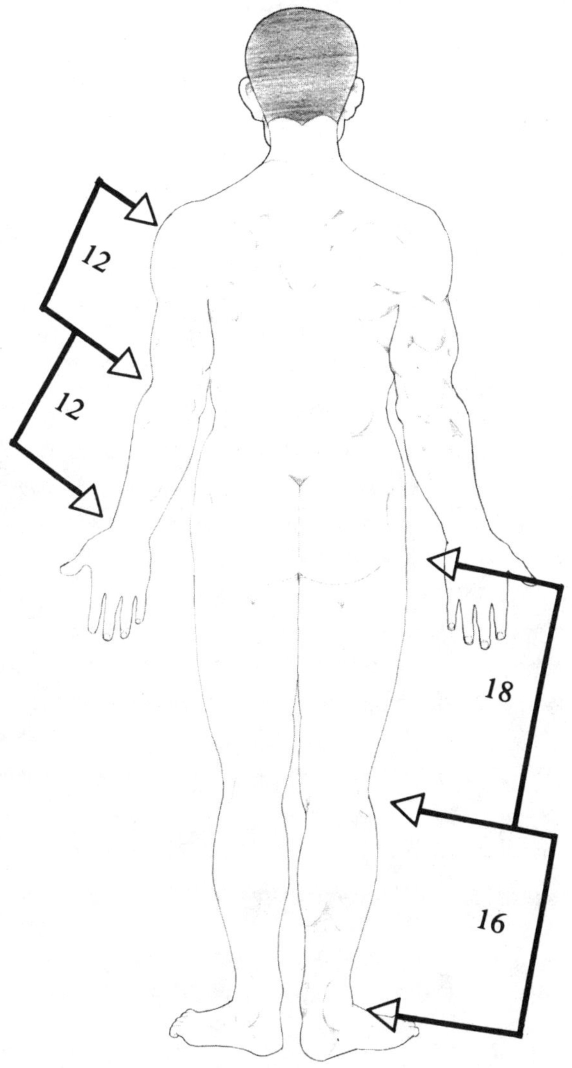

Back of Body Division Measure
Illustration 4

Acupuncture Meridians

The following are the twelve bilateral meridians of the body. The first six are on the arms, the last six are on the legs.

Acupuncture Meridians				
No.	Meridian	No. Points	Yin/Yang	Area of Body
1	Lung	11 Points	Yin	Arms
2	Heart	9 Points	Yin	Arms
3	Pericardium	9 Points	Yin	Arms
4	Large Intestine	20 Points	Yang	Arms
5	Small Intestine	19 Points	Yang	Arms
6	Triple Warmer	23 Points	Yang	Arms
7	Spleen	21 Points	Yin	Legs
8	Kidney	27 Points	Yin	Legs
9	Liver	14 Points	Yin	Legs
10	Stomach	45 Points	Yang	Legs
11	Bladder	67 Points	Yang	Legs
12	Gall Bladder	44 Points	Yang	Legs

There are two meridians along the center of the body:

Meridians along the center of the body				
1	Conception Vessel	24 Points	Yin	Front
2	Governing Vessel	28 Points	Yang	Back

All yin arm meridians flow from the center of the body to the fingertips.

All yang arm meridians flow from the fingertips to the face. (This is why the face does not easily feel cold; all the yang meridians start or end on the face.)

All yin leg meridians flow from the toes to the center of the body. All yang leg meridians flow from the face to the toes.

The Conception Vessel Meridian and Governing Vessel Meridian both flow from the center of the body up to the face, from in front of and behind the anus.

Making Division Measurments

The Division Measurement Chart on the following page, or a larger one you draw, may be used to help you correctly locate points with the aid of a "tape measure" you may construct for yourself. The following procedure should be followed.

Step	Procedure
Step One:	Chose the correct begining and ending points of the division measurement you wish to use; note the correct number of divisions.
Example:	Between the front hairline and the back hairline is twelve divisions.
Step Two:	Use paper, or a light cloth strip about an inch wide and measure the patient's body, cutting the strip to the exact length between the two anatomical landmarks.
Example:	Hold one end of a strip at the front hairline. Evenly strech the strip over the head and mark the point at which the strip crosses the back hair line. Cut at the mark.
Step Three:	Fold the strip until the folded length fits within the diagonal distance between one horizontal and one vertical mark indentified by the same number.
Example:	Since the head measurement strip won't fit on the chart fold it evenly twice creating five points: the beginning, end and three folds. The folded strip will fit evenly between the horizontal "9" and the vertical "9."
Step Four:	Use the horizontal marks to evenly space each folded section into the number of units necessary so that the total number of divisions is correct.
Example:	Divide each folded section into three even units using the "3" and "6" vertical rule.
Step Five:	This strip can be used to measure points on the patient's body. Each unit will equal one divison.

Division Measurement Chart

30													
29													
28													
27													
26													
25													
24													
23													
22													
21													
20													
19													
18													
17													
16													
15													
14													
13													
12													
11													
10													
9													
8													
7													
6													
5													
4													
3													
2													
1													
	1	2	3	4	5	6	7	8	9	10	11	12	13

Points by Area

The Points of Acupuncture

There are 360 original acupuncture points, but some of them are not often used and are therefore not as important. In this first part we will discuss the 211 most important points. This will be done by taking separate regions of the body and looking at the points in each area. In a later part, all of the points will be discussed, meridian by meridian.

Section 1 **The Points On The Head**

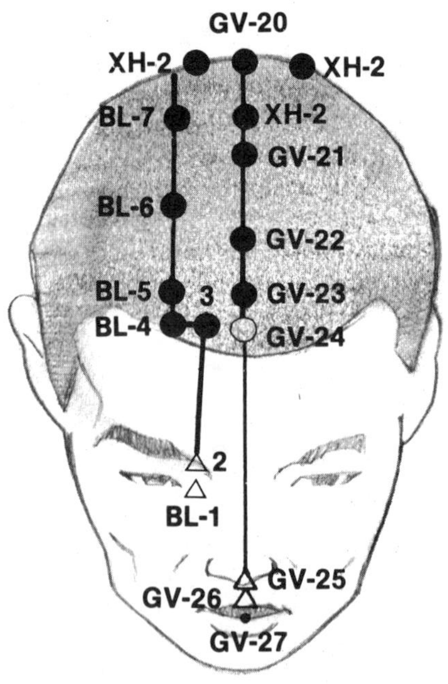

Points on the Head

Illustration 5

Center line (Governing Vessel)

1.1 **Shen Ting** *spirit courtyard* **GV-24**

Location: 1/2 division up from the front hairline; find the small hollow on the skull.

Effects: Weakness in spirit; headache (forehead); madness; convulsions; eyes weepy; chronic sinusitis; epilepsy; frightened condition and cannot sleep; dizziness; dizziness with vomiting.

Treatment: **Forbidden To Needle**, if the needle is used here it may cause madness or blindness
Moxa: 7-21 times or indirect moxa by ginger. 5 direct moxa is better, over 7 and no hair will grow again at this point.
Note: **Do not use this point at evening time**; it will prevent the patient from sleeping that whole night.

Stimulus: Acts on the center line of the forehead and lateral to the temple.

1.2 **Shang Hsing** *upper star* **GV-23**

Location: 1 division up from the front hairline.

Effects: Headache (forehead); short-sightedness; nasal polyps; purulent rhinitis; face red and swollen; face feels cold without perspiration; congestion of the face; chronic bleeding from the nose (only moxa).

Treatment: Needle: 1/8 inch deep; use the needle slanted at an angle pointing down toward the forehead.
Moxa: 5 times. Not more than 5 times, if moxa is used more than 5 times will cause dimness of the eyes.

Stimulus: Acts down on center line of the forehead.

1.3 **Shin Hui** *meeting of the skull bones* **GV-22**

Location: 2 divisions up from the front hairline. At the anterior fontanel, the soft spot where the skull bones grow together in a child.

Effects: Anemic headache; swelling of the skin on the head; epilepsy; vertigo; face pale; congestion of the face; loss of the sense of smell; convulsions in infants or children; blockage of nose; sleeps too much.

Treatment: Needle: 1/8 inch or slightly more.
Moxa: 5 times.
Warning: for children younger than 8 years old, this point is forbidden to needle or moxa.

Stimulus: Acts down toward the forehead.

1.4 **Chien Ding** *anterior summit* **GV-21**

Location: 3 and 1/2 divisions back from front hairline; also 1 and 1/2 divisions back from GV-22.

Effects: Congestion of brain; anemia of the brain; congestion of the face; swelling of the face and eyes; dizziness; headache; convulsions in children; runny nose.

Treatment: Needle: 1/8 inch deep.
Moxa: 3 to 7 times.

Stimulus: Reacts forward almost to the front hairline.

1.5 **Bai Hui** *hundred meetings* **GV-20**

Location: 5 divisions back from the front hairline in the hollow of the bone.

Effects: Headache; dizziness; heavy feeling in the head; nose bleed; nasal occlusion; cerebral hemorrhage; hemiplegia; frequent weeping; inability to choose words; epilepsy; insanity (not severe); weakness of the heart; underdevelopment of the brain in children; fear and forgetfulness; no appetite; malaria; vaginal bleeding; pre and post partum difficulties; convulsions in children; crying at night; prolapse of anus; weakness of the nerves of the entire body; anemia of the brain; congestion of the brain; chronic diarrhea; hair dropping out; gray hair at a youthful age.

Treatment: Needle: Approximately 1/8 inch.
Moxa: 3 to 5 times (not over 7 times).

Stimulus: Goes toward the four directions.

1.6 **Hou Ding** *posterior summit* **GV-19**

Location: 6 and 1/2 divisions from the front hairline, 1 and 1/2 divisions behind Bai Hui (GV-20).

Effects: Stiffness of the head and neck; occipital headache; migraine; fear of wind and cold; vertigo; epilepsy; walks around madly.

Treatment: Needle: 1/8 inch.
Moxa: 5 times.

Stimulus: Reacts down the back of the head.

Section 2 **Top of Head, Bilateral**

2.1 **Lin Chi** *temporary crying* **GB-15**

Location: On a line directly up from the pupil of the eye, 1/2 division back from the front of the hairline

Effects: Film over the eyes; excessive tears; nose blocked; congestion of outer corners of the eyes; epilepsy; convulsions in children; apoplexy.

Treatment: Needle 1/8 inch.
Moxa forbidden. If moxa is used here it will cause headache and blindness.

Stimulus: Down to the forehead as far as the eyebrow.

2.2 **Mu Chuang** *eye window* **GB-16**

Location: 2 Divisions up from front hairline, on a line directly up from the pupil of the eye.

Effects: Inflammation and pain in the eyes; unclear vision; headache; vertigo; swollen head and face; fever without perspiration; fever and chills.

Treatment: Needle: 1/8 inch.
Moxa: 5 times.

Stimulus: Down to the forehead.

Section 3 **Points Around Temples**
Points on Back of Head and Neck

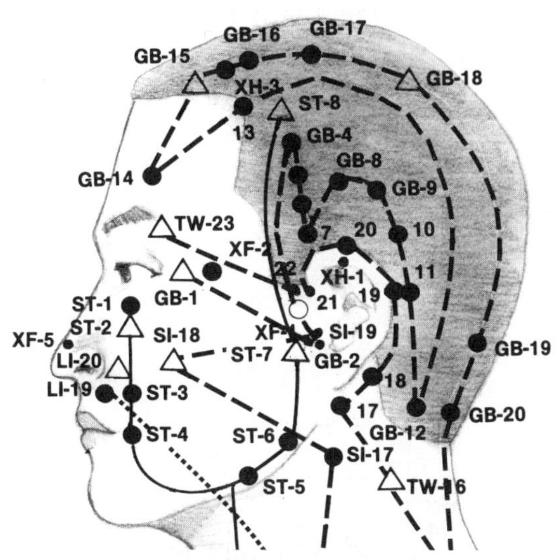

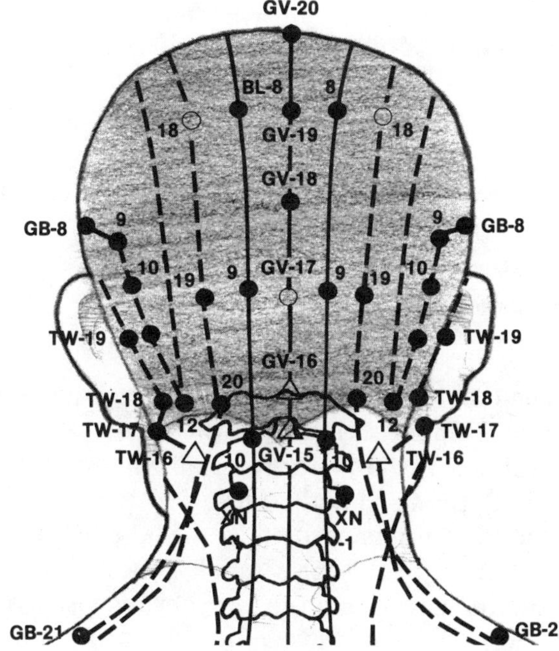

Points around the temples

Illustration 6

3.1 **Ben Shen** *natural spirit* **GB-13**

Location: On line up from the lateral end of the eyebrow, at the edge of the hair corner in the first straight, hollow cleft.

Effects: Convulsions in children; eyes dizzy; vertigo; neck stiff; madness; epilepsy; Bell's palsy; twisting of face; forehead headache.

Treatment: Needle: 1/4 inch to 1/2 inch, with the needle pointing down to the temple under the surface of the skin.
Moxa: 7 times.

Stimulus: Down to temple area.

3.2 **Tou Wee** *head binding* **ST-8**

Location: From the corner of hairline back about 1/2 division, this point is found in the third large cleft.

Effects: Headache (severe); facial paralysis; hemiplegia; numbness of the face; pain in the eyes; excessive tears; dislike of sunlight; inflammation of the eyes; blinking of the eyes; dizziness; congestion of the brain.

Treatment: Needle: 1/2 inch, point the needle toward the temple, under the surface of the skin.
No Moxa - may cause blindness.

Stimulus: Reaction down to temple area.

Note: To locate GB-13 and ST-8 slide your fingernail backward from the edge of the hair beginning in the corner of the hairline above the lateral end of the eyebrow. You will find three clefts. The first cleft is GB-13; the third and largest cleft is ST-8. The second cleft has no point but if it is needled by mistake the stimulus goes down the face in front of the ear. Usually, these three clefts are straight up from the lateral end of the eyebrow past the corner of the hairline. On some people however, the hair corner is not above the eyebrow. In this case, locate the points according to the corner of the hair only, do not use the eyebrow as a reference point.

Section 4 **Back of Head and Neck**

4.1 **Feng Fu** *wind mansion* **GV-16**

Location: 1 division up from back hairline in the hollow below occipital prominence.
Note: The point can be used as a guide, as it is 11 divisions over the midline from the point Feng Fu to the front hairline.

Effects: Apoplexy (patient cannot talk, with paralysis of tongue); epilepsy; headache; vertigo; stiffness of the neck; nose blockage; nose bleeding; throat swollen and painful; mute conditions; toothache; hallucination; delirium; fever; fear; influenza; jaundice; overheating in the chest.

Treatment: Needle: 1/3 to 1/2 inch.
No Moxa, use of moxa can cause loss of speech.
Note: While treating this point, the patient's head should remain erect.

Stimulus: Reacts upward to the two temples and down the neck towards the back, also acts forward toward the throat.

4.2 **Ya Men** *door of muteness* **GV-15**

Location: 1/2 division up from back hairline and also 1/2 division down from GV-16.

Effects: Headache; stiff neck; epilepsy; convulsions; tongue moves slowly; cannot speak; swelling of the throat; complete or partial loss of voice; nose bleeding; apoplexy; double tongue (used in addition to: LI-4, LI-11, PC-9, and a special point beneath the tongue in the veins, Jin Jin and Yu Yeh. Draw blood from the two veins bilaterlly.)

Treatment: Needle 1/3 inch to 1/2 inch deep. **No deep needle**. **No Moxa**, if moxa is used here it may cause muteness.
Note: If by mistake moxa is burnt here and causes muteness, it can be corrected if treated within 80 days as follows: direct moxa on LI-4 (1 moxa); PC-5 (2 moxa); TW-17 (3 moxa); GB-2 (1 moxa); GV-20 (2 moxa).

Stimulus: Same as Feng Fu, but does not go up to the temple.

4.3 **Tin Chu** *pillar of heaven* **BL-10**

Location: 1/2 division up from the back hairline in middle of the trapezius muscle.

Effects: Vertigo and headache; heaviness of head; stiffness of neck; cramp in neck; pain in the neck and back; legs cannot support the body; heavy feeling on the eyelids; stuffed nose with tears; weak sense of smell; torticollis.

Treatment: Needle 1/2 to 3/4 inch.
Moxa: 3-7 times.

Stimulus: Up to the temple, down to the neck and across to the shoulders.

4.4 **Feng Chi** *wind pond* **GB-20**

Location: Below the occipital bone in the hollow at the lateral edge of the trapezius muscle; this point is at the same level as Feng Fu (GV-16.)

Effects: Beginning of influenza attack (feels cold with fever and no sweating); sunstroke; migraine; after apoplexy when phlegm comes from the mouth and the patient cannot speak (this is a dangerous condition); dizziness; stiffness of neck; weakness of brain; headache in the whole head and/or occipital region; eyes dizzy and vision unclear; excessive tears; wind causing the eyes to water; inflammation of the eyes; night blindness; nose bleed; nose blocked; runny nose; tinnitus; partial deafness; back painful; weakness of the neck or lack of energy in the neck when the patient cannot straighten their neck (use moxa).

Treatment: Needle 1/2 to 1 inch deep according to the size of the patient.
Moxa: 3-7 times.

Stimulus: Up to the temple and down to the base of the neck.

Section 5 **Area Around The Ear**

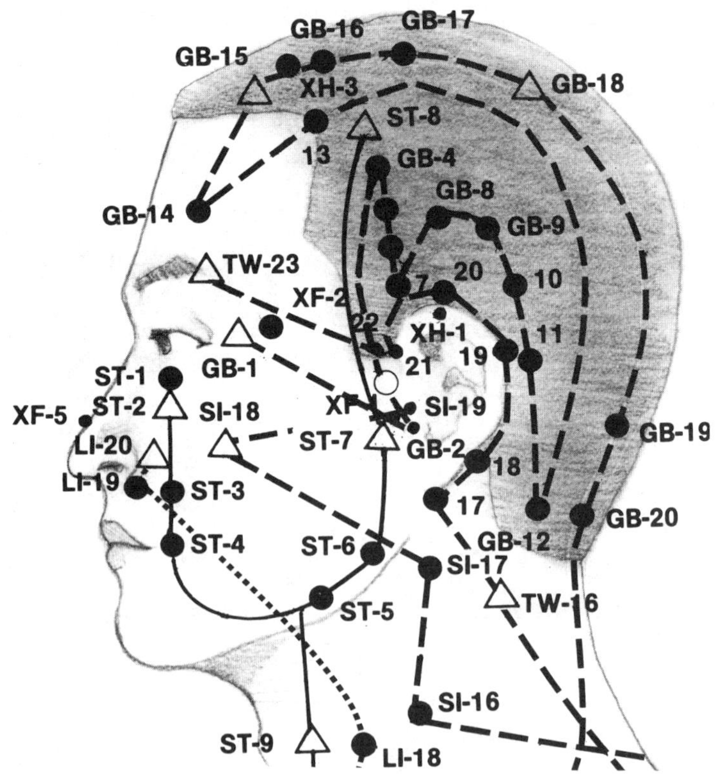

Area Around The Ear

Illustration 7

5.1 **Er Men** *ear door* **TW-21**

Location: Out 1/3 division from the gap between the tragus and the helix between the ear and the jaw bone. Try to open the mouth, there is a hollow there.

Effects: Ringing in the ear; deafness; inflammation of the ear (otitis media); pain of the inner ear; fluid coming from the ear; toothache of the upper jaw; lips stiff; abcess in the ear.

Treatment: Needle: 1/4 inch deep.
Moxa: 3 times.

Stimulus: Inward to the ear and upward to the temple.

Note: At this point there is a pulse; one must be careful with the needle. Use your finger to find the pulse. If the pulse is a little above the point, use the fingernail to pull the pulse upward and insert the needle below the fingernail. If the pulse is a little lower than the point, use the same method to pull the pulse down and insert the needle above the fingernail. If the pulse is right on the middle of the point, one must be very careful.

5.2 **Ting Hui** *meeting of hearing* **GB-2**

Location: Out 1/3 eye division horizontally from the "V" formed by the tragus and the earlobe, in the crossing hollow of the jaw bone

Effects: Deafness; ringing in the ear; inflammation of the middle ear; paralysis of one side of face (Bell's Palsy); slackness of the jaw bone; cramping of the jaw muscles.

Treatment: Needle: 1/4 inch deep, up to touching the bone.
Moxa: 3-5 times.

Stimulus: Inward to the ear and across to the face and jaw.

5.3 **Ting Gung** *palace of listening* **SI-19**

Location: Out from center of the tragus, 1/3 division, in the crossing hollow of the bone (horizontal cleft).

Effects: Deafness; tinnitus; inflammation of the ear; blockage of the ear.

Treatment: Needle: 1/4 inch deep, up to touching the bone.
Moxa: 3 times.

Stimulus: Inward to the ear, across to the face ending below the nose.

5.4 **Yi Fung** *wind block* **TW-17**

Location: Behind the bottom of the ear lobe just behind the jaw bone.

Effects: Deafness; tinnitus; slackness of jaw; cramping of jaw; paralysis of face; hiccough; mumps; scrofula; chronic yawning in infants.

Treatment: Needle: 1/2 inch; during treatment the patient should open their mouth about 1/4 inch wide.
Moxa: 3 to 7 times.

Stimulus: Inward to the ear, downward to the neck.

Note: The preceeding four points (TW-21, GB-2, SI-19 and TW-17) are used for deafness. The patient must open the mouth very wide during insertion; the needles are inserted deeply (over 1 inch) and left in place for one-half hour.

5.5 **Jia Che** *chariot of the jaw* **ST-6**

Location: Above the angle of the jaw bone, 1/3 division up from the edge of the jaw bone in the hollow of the masseter muscle, 1/4 division anterior to the edge of the jaw bone.

Effects: Swelling of the jaw; cramping of the jaw after a stroke; cannot speak; paralysis of the facial muscles; stiffness of neck; slackness of the jaw; trigeminal neuralgia; toothache of the lower jaw.

Treatment: Needle 1/4 inch.
Moxa: 3 times.

Stimulus: Up to the ear and down to the lower jaw and mouth.

Section 6 **Area Around the Eyes**

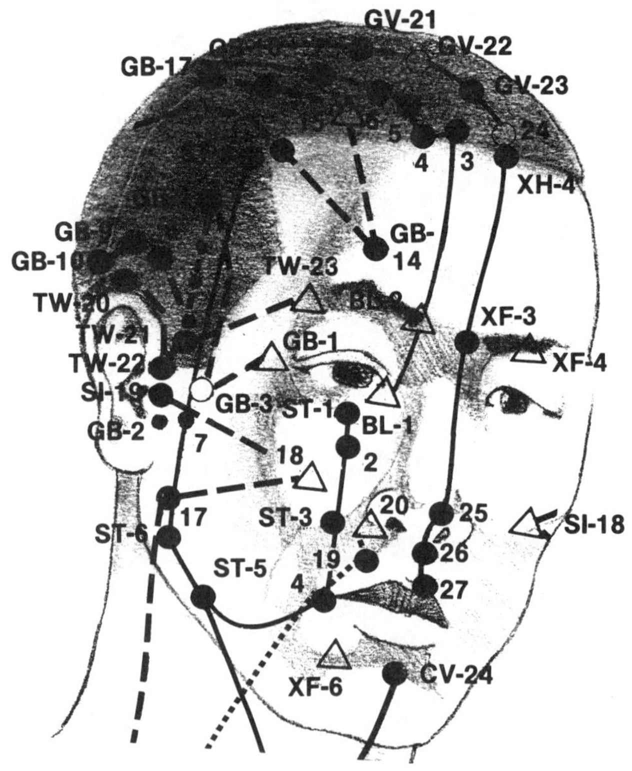

Area around the Eyes
Illustration 8

6.1 **Yang Bai** *yang white* **GB-14**

Location: About one division above the middle of the eyebrow and about 1/2 division lateral in a small hollow. One can feel the nerve with the finger. On high foreheads the point is about 3/4 of a division up from the eyebrow.

Effects: Itching in the eyes; poor night vision; eyes locked looking up; eyes twitch; eyes red and swollen; headache in the forehead; myopia; pain in the eyes; coldness of the body.

Treatment: Needle 1/5 inch deep.
Moxa: 3 times.

Stimulus: Goes vertically up the forehead to one side of the top of the head.

6.2 **Ts'uan Jhu** *drilling bamboo* **BL-2**

Location: At the medial end of the eyebrow, in the hollow.

Effects: Madness; eyes red and painful with headache; itching in eyes; eyes lazy; eye wanders; vision foggy; excessive tearing with dizziness; convergent strabismus; pain in the eyebrow; pain in the forehead; hay fever; allergic rhinorrhea; sinusitis; supraorbital neuralgia; hallucinations; nightmares; night blindness; white spot on the iris.
For inflammation of the eyes use a prismatic needle and draw out several drops of blood.

Treatment: Needle 1/5 to 1/4 inch deep.
No Moxa.

Stimulus:
1) Going toward the other eyebrow.
2) Going laterally to the outside of the eyebrow.
3) Going up to the forehead.
4) Going down to the nose with a little electric feeling.

Note: There is a small pulse at this point.

6.3 **Si-Jhu Kung** *silk bamboo hollow* **TW-23**

Location: In the hollow at the lateral end of the eyebrow. Some eyebrows are long, others are short.

Effects: White spots on the iris; eyes locked staring up; temple headaches; eyes red, swollen and painful; eyes twitching or blinking separately; facial paralysis; convulsions in children; optic atrophy; blurred vision; tears flow in bright light; vomiting of excessive saliva and mucus with madness; dizziness.

Treatment: Needle 1/10 to 1/5 inch.
No Moxa.

Stimulus: Reaction to the temple area.
Note: There is a small pulse at this point.

6.4 **Jing Ming** *eye bright* **BL-1**

Location: 1/10 inch out from the medial canthus of the eye.

Effects: Eye disease; eyes dizzy; inner canthus red and painful; conjunctivitis; tears flow in wind; dim vision; retinitis; poor night vision; eyelid dropping down; muscle-like vasculature growing from canthus to iris (pterygium).

Treatment: Needle: 1/10 inch to 2/10 inch. There is a small muscle ball visible in the medial canthus; the needle should be inserted at the medial side of this ball (the side closest to the nose) and also on the center line of the muscle ball.
No Moxa.

Stimulus: Running around the entire eyeball with a slight electric feeling.

Note: There is a small pulse at this point.

6.5 **Tung-Tzi Liao** *bone hole of eye* **GB-1**

Location: 1/2 eye division lateral from external canthus on the orbital bone.

Effects: Headaches; color blindness; night blindness; optic atrophy; outer corners of eye red and swollen; myopia; retinal hemorrhage; conjunctivitis; keratitis; trigeminal neuralgia; paralysis of the face.

Treatment: Needle: 1/10 inch.
No Moxa.

Stimulus: 1) On one side going towards the eye.
2) On the other side going towards the temple.

Section 7 **Points Around the Nose**

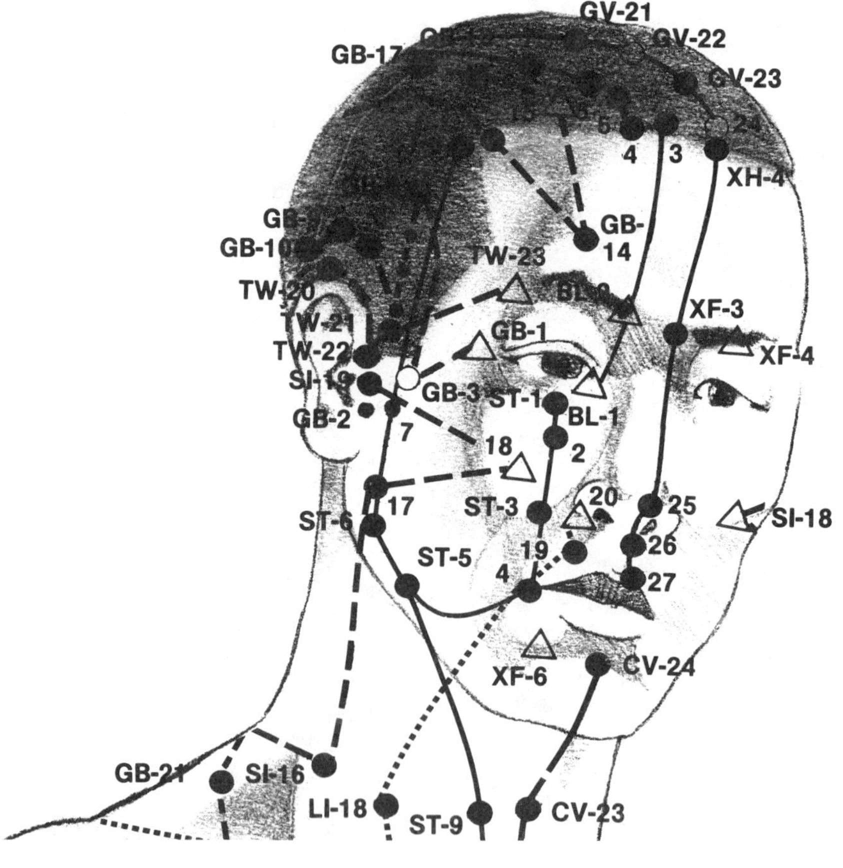

Points around the Nose
Illustration 9

7.1 **Su Liao** *pure white bone hole* **GV-25**

Location: At the straight cleft on the center of the tip of the nose.

Effects: Nose congestion; polyps; bulbous nose from excessive drinking; epistaxis; running nose; stuffed nose.

Treatment: Needle: 1/2 inch or a little less. This point is painful to treat. With red, bulbous nose, use prismatic needle, draw out 3-4 drops of blood.
No Moxa.

Stimulus: Throughout the entire nose with tears from the eyes.

7.2 **Ying Hsiang** *accept fragrance* **LI-20**

Location: 1/2 eye division from outer side of nostril on the "smile line" at the level of the bottom of the nostril.

Effects: Nose catarrh; stuffed nose; anosmia; rhinorrhea; facial paralysis; nasal polyps; epistaxis; swollen face; itching on the face; numbness with the feeling of insects crawling under the skin (combine with GV-26); sounds during breathing; swollen lips.

Treatment: Needle: 1/8 to 1/4 inch.
No Moxa.

Stimulus: Up to the nostril; often down to the gums.

Section 8 **Points Around the Mouth**

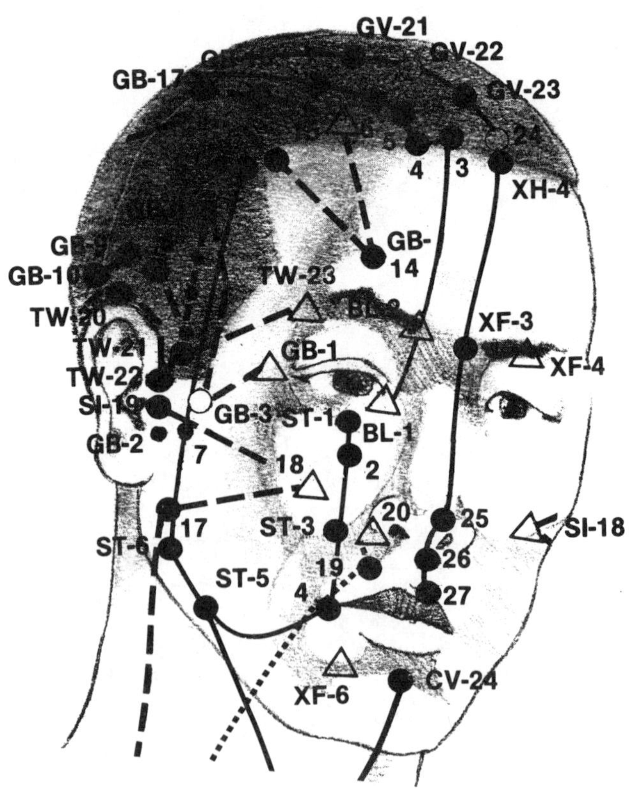

Points around the Mouth

Illustration 10

8.1 **Shui Kou** *water ditch*

Ren Jung *middle of man* **GV-26**

Location: In the center of the philtrum; some charts and books show this point a little higher than the middle. In my experience this is not correct.

Effects: Fainting; apoplexy; delirium; epilepsy; madness; hysteria; eclampsia; edema of the face; excessive thirst; toothache of the upper jaw; heat stroke; lumbago; pain along vertebral column; swollen face with a feeling of insects crawling in the skin; poor eyesight; convulsions; cramping and twitching of the eye or mouth; dizziness and fainting after needling.

Treatment: Needle: 1/8 to 1/4 inch.
No Moxa, if moxa is used here the patient will die.

Stimulus: Painful, with tears running and saliva coming from mouth.

8.2 **Ti T'sang** *earth granary* **ST-4**

Location: 4/10 of an eye division lateral to the edge of mouth.

Effects: Neuralgia and paralysis of the face; lockjaw; toothache; swollen jaw; cannot close eyelid or blink; acute dumbness; inability to speak; laryngitis; night blindness; nystagmus; itching in the eye; for relaxing tight muscles of the face.

Treatment: Needle: 1/8 to 1/4 inch.
Moxa: 5 times.

Stimulus: Slight local stimulus around the corners of the mouth.

8.3 **Cheng Jiang** *receiving starch* **CV-24**

Location: In the depression between the point of the chin and the lower lip, on the line of the Conception Vessel.

Effects: Paralysis of the face; numbness of the face; lockjaw; thirst; swelling of the face; toothache; pain of dental caries; dental abscess in gums; acute dumbness.

Treatment: Needle: 1/8 to 1/4 inch (to treat, open the mouth 1/4 inch).
Moxa: 7 times.

Stimulus: Reaction goes to lower lip; inside to gums and teeth and saliva comes out of the mouth.

Section 9 **Special Points on Head and Neck**

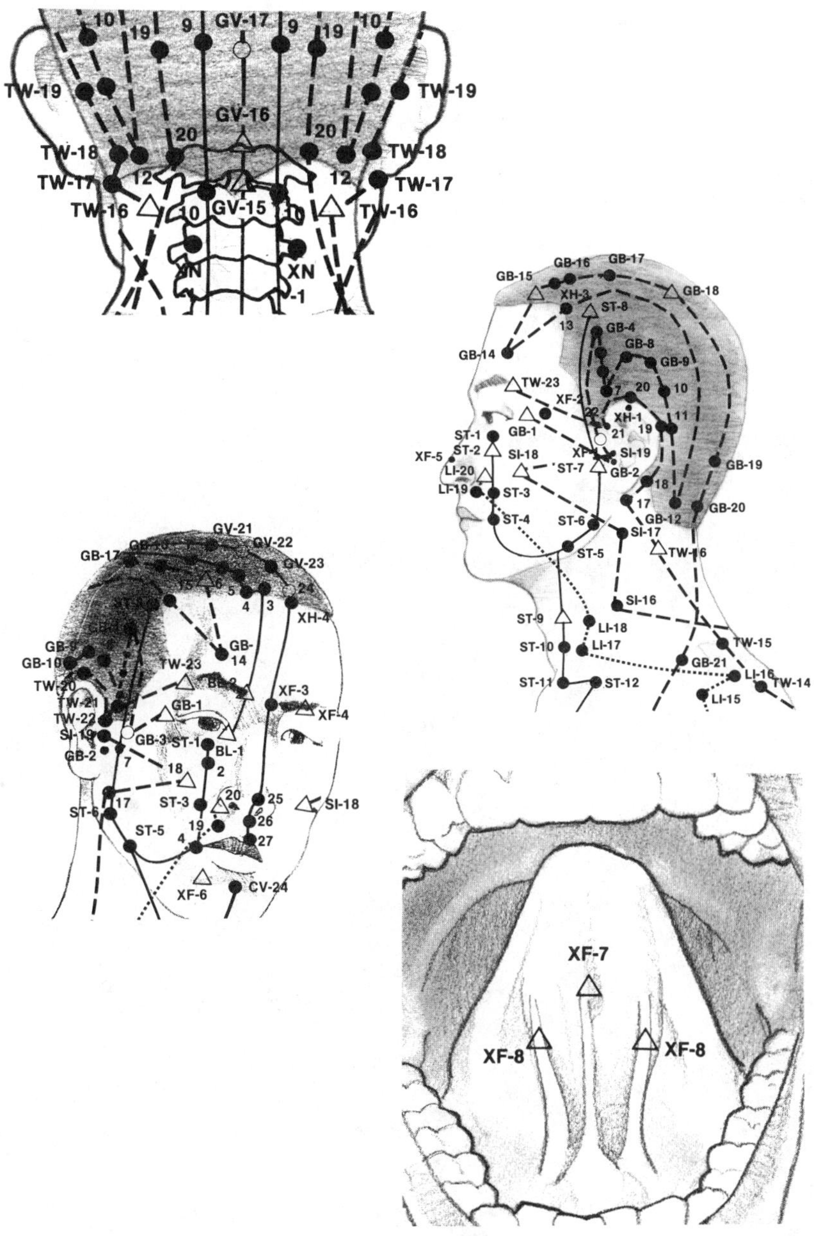

Special points on the Head and Neck

Illustration 11

9.1 **Pak Loh** *one hundred labors* **XN-1**

Location: Down 1/3 of the distance between the back hairline and the seventh cervical vertebrae. Out from the midline one eye division. From the back hairline to the seventh cervical vertebrae is divided into 3 divisions. When locating this point the neck should be straight up.

Effects: Scrofula; goiter; stiffness of the neck.

Treatment: For goiter and stiffness of the neck, needle 1/4 to 3/4 inch.
For scrofula use only direct moxa 7 times.

Stimulus: Up to the back of the head, down to the bottom of the neck. Insertion to 3/4 inch depth stimulates inward to the thyroid.

9.2 **Er Jen** *upper point of ear* **XH-1**

Location: Fold the outer ear, this point is at the top of the sharp point formed by the fold.

Effects: Film over the eye (beginning stages); cloudy urine; discharge in women.

Treatment: **No Needle.**
Moxa: the size of 1/2 rice grain, 5 to 7 times.

Stimulus: Up to the hair area and down to the bottom of the ear.

9.7 **Tai Yang** *solar* **XF-2**

Location: Between the eyebrow and the outer canthus of the eye, going back one eye division, where there is a crossing cleft.

Effects: Migraine headache; inflammation of the eyeball.

Treatment: Needle: 1/2 to 1 inch.
Moxa: 3 times.
Note: Use the needle for inflammation of the eyeball and migraine from an overheating condition. You can also remove a few drops of blood from the vein in this area. For overcooling conditions use 3 moxa after the needle.

Stimulus: The reaction is felt around the inside of the whole temple area.
Note: A pulse is close to this point; before treatment find the pulse.

9.8 **Yin Tang** *hall of seal* **XF-3**

Location: On the Governing Vessel line between the two eyebrows.

Effects: Convulsions in children; headaches; dizziness; vertigo; local pain; dizziness from excessive uterine bleeding after childbirth; vomiting; nose blocked.

Treatment: Needle: 1/8 inch.
Moxa: 5 times.

Stimulus: Up to the forehead; down to the nose and across to both eyebrows.

9.9 **Yu Yao** *fish loins* **XF-4**

Location: In the depression in the middle of the eyebrow.

Effects: Conjunctivitis; dropping of eyelid.

Treatment: For dropping of eyelid insert the needle a short distance, 1/8 inch; get the stimulus and then while lifting up the skin, direct the needle towards the medial end of the eyebrow (towards BL-2). Then, get the stimulus, raise the needle and direct it towards the lateral end of the eyebrow (towards TW-23) and get the stimulus again.
No Moxa.

Stimulus: Local stimulus.

9.10 **Pie Yen** *eyes of the nose* **XF-5**

Location: Lateral to the midline and midpoint of the nose, between the hard and soft bones at the top of the triangular corner.

Effects: All nose problems.

Treatment: Needle: less than 1/8 inch.
No Moxa.

Stimulus: Light electrical stimulus through the whole nostril.

9.11 **Jia-Cheng Jiang** *beside receiving starch* **XF-6**

Location: One eye division lateral to CV-24.

Effects: Epidemic, frog head epidemic; swelling of the face; furuncle on lips.

Treatment: Needle: about 1/4 inch. One can use the prismatic needle to draw several drops of blood.
No Moxa.

Stimulus: Towards each side of the chin.

9.12 **Hai Chuen** *sea spring* **XF-7**

Location: Under the tongue, on the midline, about 1/16 inch up from the vinculum lingua.

Effects: Excessive thirst; burning sensation in the center of the chest.

Treatment: Use the needle for shallow insertion, 1/8 inch, and draw out a little blood. Do not use the prismatic needle, use a thicker acupuncture needle.
No Moxa.

Stimulus: Local stimulus, only a little painful.

9.13 **Jin Jin (left)** *golden fluid* and 9.14 **Yu-Yeh (right)** *jade fluid* XF-8

Location: On the veins, on both sides of the vinculum lingua, when the tongue is rolled up.

Effects: Excessive thirst; tongue swollen and painful; abcess in the mouth; aphasia; flame or hot sensation in chest (see: Hai-Chuen XF-7); morning sickness.

Treatment: Shallow insertion to cause bleeding. Use a thicker needle and pricking technique, not a prismatic needle.
No Moxa.

Stimulus: A little local pain.

Section 10 **Neck and Chest Area**

Center line of the Body

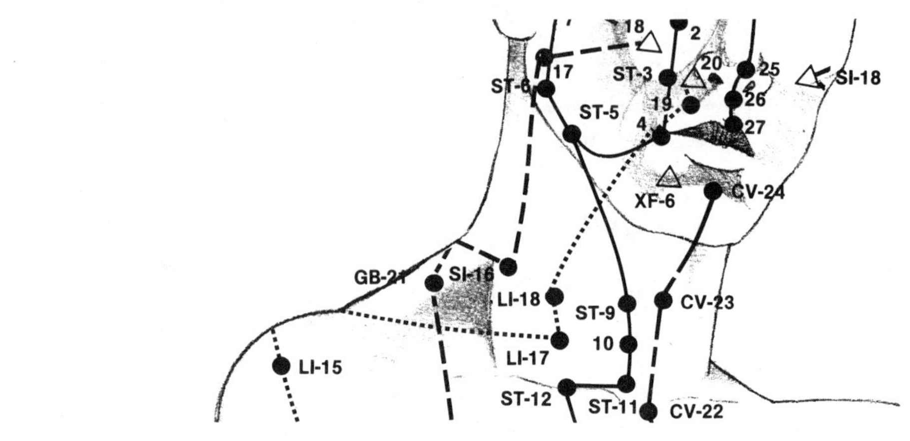

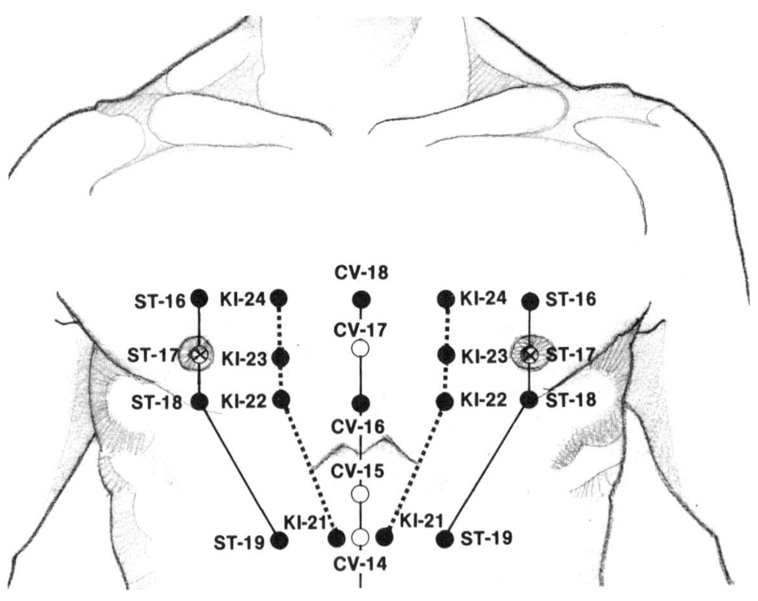

Neck and Chest Area

Illustration 12

10.1 **Lien Ch'uan** *pure spring* **CV-23**

Location: Upon the Adam's apple in the hollow of the "V." On females this bone is a little high and small.

Effects: Bronchitis; dyspnea; pharyngitis; vomiting; swelling of the tongue; hacking cough; tongue loose; tongue stiff; dribbling of saliva; double tongue; dumbness; catarrh from the bronchus; abcess in the mouth.

Treatment: Needle: 1/4 to 3/8 inch.
Moxa: 3 times.
Note: The head should be raised a little, not too high or the point will disappear. Warn the patient not to talk or swallow during insertion or while the needle is in the skin.

Stimulus: Reaction is felt in the throat under the tongue, like a fish bone in the throat.

10.2 **T'ien T'u** *heavenly rushing* **CV-22**

Location: Located on the anterior median line of the neck, at the top of the sternum bone, in the hollow behind the bone.

Effects: Dyspnea; bronchitis; asthma; hemoptysis (coughing up blood from the lungs); dry cough; noise in the throat like the sound of a bird; throat swollen; stenosis of the esophagus; dumbness; aphonia; esophageal spasm; glottis spasm; stiff tongue; goiter; vomiting; hiccoughs; face feeling hot; pain from the chest connecting with the back making breathing difficult; abcess in the larynx.

Treatment: Needle: 1/2 inch or 1 and 1/2 inch.
Moxa: 3 to 5 times.

Stimulus: When the needle is inserted 1/2 inch, the stimulus will be felt around the throat and tonsil like a fishbone in the throat. When the needle is inserted 1 and 1/2 inches, the stimulus will run up the outer sides of the thyroid gland to the jaw, and down the midline of the sternum. The needle is inserted at a 75 degree angle, up to down, for both depths of insertion.

10.3 **Shin-Jung, Tang Jung**

in the middle of the fat **CV-17**

Location: At the height of both nipples upon the median line. Note: For people with curved ribs, you should follow the fourth intercostal space to the sternum; the point will be higher than the level of the two nipples. For women with heavy breasts, follow the fifth intercostal space from Yu-Ken (ST-18) toward the sternum, then jump up one rib to the center of the sternum to locate CV-17.

Effects: Dyspnea; insufficient lactation; coughing; hematemesis; hemoptysis; heart and chest painful; asthma; emphysema; belching; stenosis of the esophagus; cancer in esophagus; vomiting with phlegm and pus; cancer of breast in the first stage.

Treatment: **No Needle.**
Moxa: 7 times. The patient should be lying face up on the table when applying moxa.

Stimulus: Spreads over the whole chest area.

10.4 **Jung Ting** *middle courtyard* **CV-16**

Location: One rib bone below Shin-Jung (CV-17), at the fifth intercostal space; directly across from ST-18 on the midline.

Effects: Lung congestion; chest and ribs swollen and painful; dyspnea; tonsillitis; vomiting; vomiting of milk by children; stenosis of the esophagus.

Treatment: Needle: 1/4 to 1/2 inch.
Moxa: 3 to 5 times.

Stimulus: Down to the stomach.

Section 11 **Chest and Flank Area**

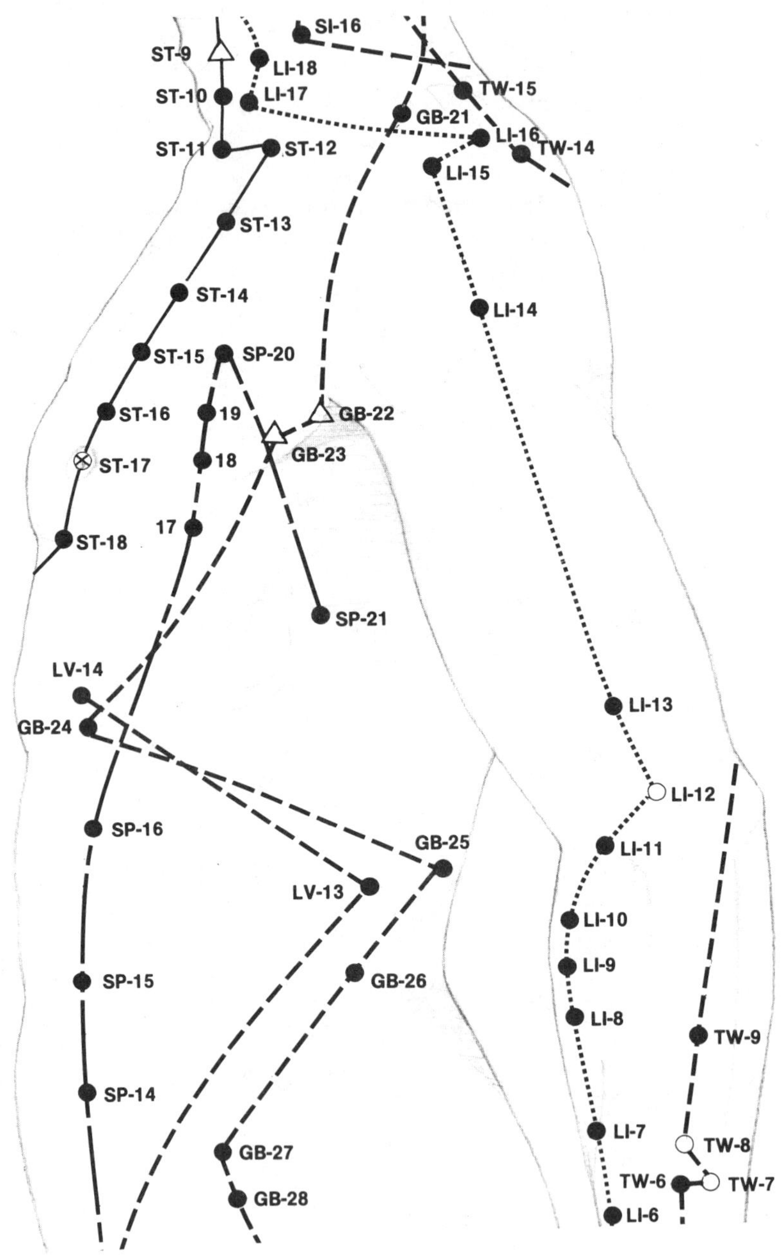

Chest and Flank area

Illustration 13

11.1 **Ch'ueh Pen** *broken basin* **ST-12**

Location: Behind the middle of the superior border of the clavicle, vertically above the nipple, four divisions from the middle line of the trunk.

Effects: Incessant coughing; chest feeling hot and full with difficulty in breathing; local intercostal neuralgia; inflammation of throat; scrofula; pleurisy.

Treatment: Needle: 1/4 to 1/2 inch.
Moxa: 3 times.
Note: There is a pulse at this point; find the pulse before inserting the needle.

Stimulus: Down to the chest.

11.2 **Ying Chuang** *chest window* **ST-16**

Location: One rib space directly above nipple.

Effects: Ulcer or carbuncle of breast; cancer inside the breast; shortness of breath; emphysema; intercostal neuralgia; fever with sensation of cold; swelling of the ribs; burning feeling in the chest.

Treatment: Needle: 1/4 to 3/8 inch.
Moxa: 5 times.

Stimulus: Felt moving inside the whole breast.

11.3 **Ru Gun** *root of breast* **ST-18**

Location: One rib directly below the nipple in the 5th intercostal space.

Effects: Mastitis; carbuncle or cancer in the breast; pleurisy; intercostal pain and numbness; full feeling in the chest with pain; cramping during cholera; swelling and pain in the arms; hacking cough; hiccough; not enough milk for breastfeeding.

Treatment: Needle: 1/4 to 3/8 inch.
Moxa: 5 times.

Stimulus: Felt moving inside the whole breast.

11.4 **Chi Men** *waiting door* **LV-14**

Location: Up from the umbilicus six divisions and across from the midline four divisions; in between two ribs, between the sixth and seventh rib bones.

Effects: After the flu, a feeling of overheating in the chest; pains in the heart; asthma such that the patient cannot sleep or sit; vomiting sour tasting vomit; food and drink cannot descend the digestive tract; vomiting of stomach fluid after eating; mouth dry and very thirsty; chest and abdomen swollen with gas where you can feel the gas under the rib cage and it can move up and down; intercostal neuralgia; hepatitis; pleurisy; peritonitis; diarrhea; cholera; difficult delivery; post-partum troubles such as hiccoughs and belching.

Treatment: Needle: 1/4 inch or a little more.
Moxa: 5 times; for post-partum troubles, apply 5 direct moxa. If a woman feels pain in the vagina during intercourse, moxa this point and BL-23.

Stimulus: Reaction up the mammary line, over the nipple.

Note: There are two extremes to the shape of the rib cage. One is a normal "A" shape; the other is a flatter "A" shape. For the normal

"A" shape, this point would follow the above measurements. For the flatter "A" shape, according to the preceding measurements, the point would not fall between two rib bones. For this kind of shape, continue laterally until arriving between the two rib bones, this will be the correct point.

Rib Cage shapes

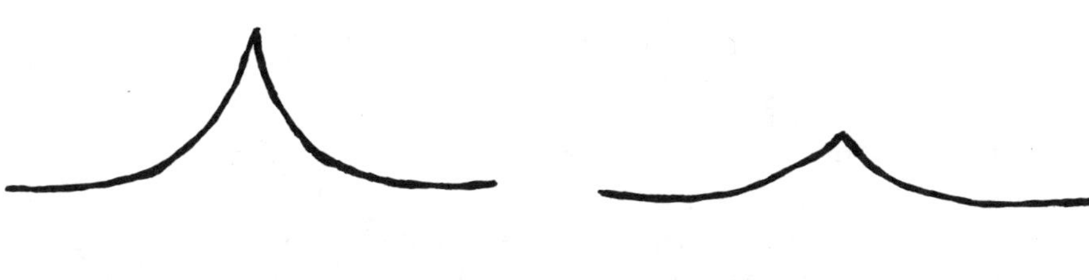

Normal *"A"* shape　　Flatter *"A"* shape

11.5 **Chung Fu** *middle mansion* **LU-1**

Location: Across from the center line 6 divisions, between the second and third rib, six divisions lateral from the center line.

Effects: A feeling of hotness in the chest during the flu; panting with a sensation of a full chest; coughing and cannot lie down; tonsillitis; swelling on the face and arms; pain on the shoulder and back; pleurisy; pneumonia; asthma; tuberculosis; tumor on skin; swelling of the four limbs.

Treatment: Needle 1/4 to 1/2 inch.
Moxa: 5 times.
Note: Needling at this point can take away all overheating in the chest.

Stimulus: Reaction down to the upper part of the chest.

11.6 **Jang Men** *seal door* **LV-13**

Location: Up two divisions from the umbilicus, across 6 divisions, just below the end of the 11th rib.
Note: for fat bellies, six divisions across falls short of the 11th rib; for women with big chests and small waists six divisions across passes the 11th rib. For these patients, locate the point as just in front (1/4 inch) of the 11th rib.

Effects: Gas inside at both sides of the body just above the waist such that the skin outside is hard as stone; swelling of the abdomen with sounds coming from inside the intestines; indigestion; vomiting; diarrhea; chest and ribs painful, patient cannot lie down or turn over; pleurisy; hepatitis; panting; pain in the heart area; swelling of the abdomen with gas; swelling of the spleen (moxa); four limbs tired; cannot raise up the arms; chronic malaria (moxa); constipation. This is a special point for any disease of the five solid organs.

Treatment: Needle: 1/4 to 1/2 inch.
Moxa: 5 to 10 times.

Stimulus: Up to the ribs, down to the belly.

11.7 **Dai Mo** *waistband pulse* **GB-26**

Location: Across from the umbilicus 8 divisions, at the same level as the umbilicus, on the midaxillary line, at the top of the iliac crest.
Note: For fat or thin bodies, disregard the 8 divisions part of this measurement.

Effects: Red or white vaginal discharge; uterine prolapse; lower quadrant pain; false urge to bowel movement due to pelvic pressure; irregular menses; pain in the uterus; pain in the upper part of the hips, radiating down the abdomen; dysmenorrhea (irregular menses).

Treatment: Needle: 1/2 to 3/4 inch.
Moxa: 5 times.

Stimulus: From the top of the iliac crest down to center of lower abdomen.

Section 12 **Upper Abdomen, Center Line**

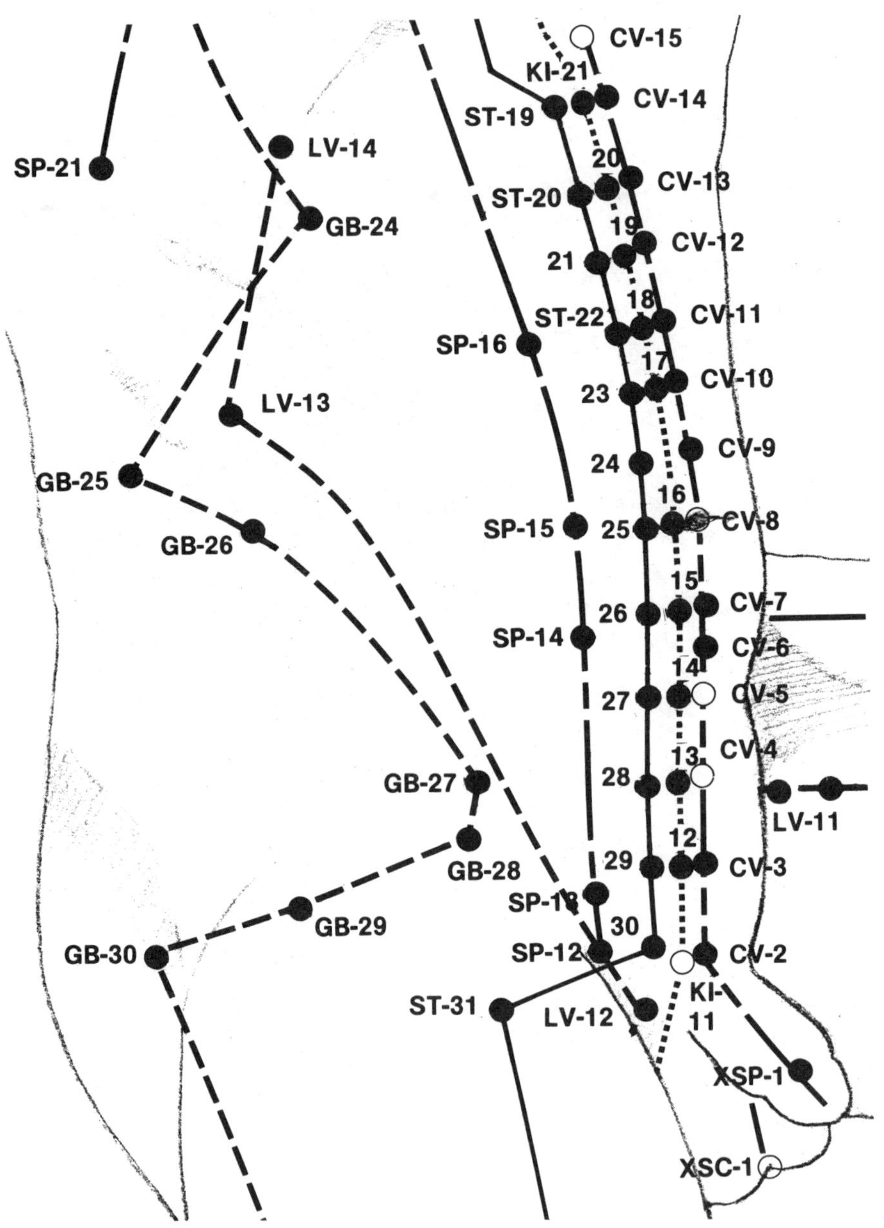

Upper Abdomen
Illustration 14

Upper Abdomen

From the xiphoid process to the pubic bone on the center line lies a hair line (a line of hair organized vertically in the midline of the body). In Chinese people you can also find a color line, a line darker in color than the rest of the skin. Underneath this line is a nerve. By touching with your fingertip you can feel the soft string of the nerve. A needle inserted on this line should touch the nerve to get the correct stimulation. For patients with a lot of fatty tissue, you must completely penetrate fatty tissue before you will be able to touch the muscle tissue and the nerve. The needle will feel relatively loose when penetrating the fatty tissue, and relatively tighter when it does touch the muscle. After touching the muscle tissue, penetrate a little deeper and you will be able to find the correct stimulation.

12.1 **Chiu Wei** *turtledove tail* **CV-15**

Location: One division below the xiphoid process, seven divisions above the umbilicus. It is eight divisions from the umbilicus to the xiphoid process, not seven, as is shown on many charts.

Effects: Palpitations of the heart; inflammmation of the pericardium; epilepsy; madness; foolishness; cerebral weakness; angina pectoris; gastric pain; chest full with coughing and vomiting; throat swollen and fluid does not descend; hemoptysis; feeling of hatred for human noise (use in conjunction with ST-44).

Treatment: **No Needle** (needle would shorten life).
Moxa: 3-5 times.

Stimulus: Up the midline of the chest and inside to the heart.

12.2 **Jiuh Chueh** *great palace gate* **CV-14**

Location: Up from the umbilicus six divisions, on the center line.

Effects: Chest full with coughing and short breathing; chest painful; cardiac pain; vomiting; swollen upper abdomen; jaundice; cramping in the diaphragm; cramping in the upper abdominal region; madness; hernia; shortness of breath walking up the stairs.

Treatment: Needle: 1/4 to 1/2 inch; no deep needle.
Moxa: 5 times.

Stimulus: Up the center line, inside to chest.

12.3 **Shang Goan** *upper stomach* **CV-13**

Location: Five divisions up from umbilicus on the center line.

Effects: Palpitations of the heart; chest feels hot and painful; peritonitis; pain in the stomach; a hard mass in abdomen (like a dish); cholera; indigestion; gas inside of the stomach area; jaundice; epilepsy; vomiting blood (hematemesis); vomiting with phlegm.

Treatment: Needle: 1/2 to 3/4 inch.
Moxa: 5 times.

Stimulus: Up the center line to the xiphoid process.

12.4 **Jung Goan** *middle stomach* **CV-12**

Location: Up from the umbilicus four divisions on the center line.

Effects: All stomach disorders; enlargement of the stomach; cramping in the stomach; bleeding from the stomach; cancer of the stomach; inflammation of the stomach; anorexia; food difficult to digest; acute gastroenteritis; diarrhea; cholera; both the heart and stomach painful; abdomen swollen like a drum; jaundice; epilepsy; dropsy; dysentery with white or red color; constipation.

Treatment: Needle: 1/2 to 3/4 inch.
Moxa: 7 times.

Stimulus: Felt locally, within a diameter of one to two inches.

12.5 **Chien Li** *established mile* **CV-11**

Location: Three divisions up from the umbilicus.

Effects: Abdomen swollen and painful; spasm in the lower abdomen; vomiting; anorexia; poor digestion; cardiac pain with the sensation of energy moving up to the chest.

Treatment: Needle: 1/2 inch or a little more.
Moxa: 5 times. **Warning: No Moxa During Pregnancy.**

Stimulus: Around the point, not as wide an area as CV-12.

12.6 **Shia Goan** *lower stomach* **CV-10**

Location: Two divisions up from the umbilicus.

Effects: Abdomen painful; abdomen distended; vomiting; anorexia; tumor in the abdomen (moxa); food not digested; gradual emaciation; abdomen swollen like a drum; stomachache; gastritis; gastric spasm; dilation of the stomach.

Treatment: Needle: 1/2 inch or a little more.
Moxa: 5 times. For tumor of the abdomen, use moxa on this point a total of 100 times, starting with 27 times each day until a total of 100 times is reached.

Stimulus: Around the area of the point.

12.7 **Shui Fen** *divided water* **CV-9**

Location: One division above the umbilicus.

Effects: Edema; ascites; pain around the umbilicus; poor appetite; enlargement of the stomach; pain or cramp in the lumbar vertebrae; fontanel does not close in a child (apply direct moxa here and CV-7.)

Treatment: Needle: 1/2 to 3/4 inch.
Moxa: 49 to 400 times, generally 5 times.

Stimulus: Reaction down to urethra.

12.8 **Shen Chueh** *God's palace gate* **CV-8**

Location: In the center of the umbilicus.

Effects: Unconscious from apoplexy; edema; swelling of the abdomen; a sound like flowing water in the intestines; cholera; a cold feeling in the whole belly; diarrhea; epilepsy in children; dysentery in children; anuria with swelling of the bladder; rectal prolapse; any disease of the stomach or intestines; visceroptosis; gastroptosis; incessant lactation and dripping of milk; miscarriage. If a woman has a history of miscarriages, before or after conception, apply moxa on this point to help protect the child. Use 30 yellow soybean size moxa. If during sexual intercourse a man cannot hold his ejaculation such that the semen runs out uncontrolably (this is called losing the yang), apply 10 soybean size moxa on CV-8 to save his life.

Treatment: **No Needle.**
Note: The old book says, if you apply a needle to the umbilicus an ulcer will form, and the faeces will come out through the umbilicus and the patient will die.
Moxa: 3-100 times.
Note: If the umbilicus is deep, fill with salt to the level of the rest of the abdomen, and apply moxa on the salt. If the umbilicus is flat, burn directly on the skin. After applying the moxa, a blister will form; don't pierce the blister, let it dry up on its own. If the blister breaks, clean off the liquid and apply mercurochrome.

Stimulus: Down to the urethra, and up to the stomach.

Section 13 **Lower Abdomen, Center Line**

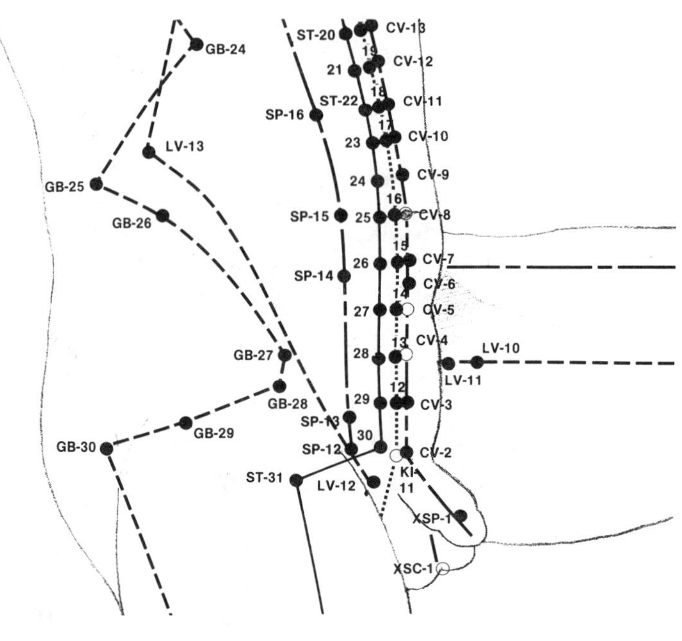

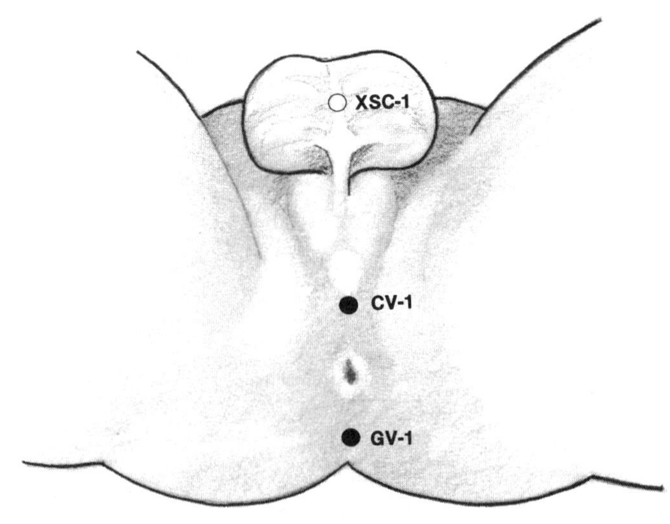

Lower Abdomen
Illustration 15

13.1 **Yin Jiao** *yin transfer* **CV-7**

Location: One division below the center of the umbilicus. Note: From the center of the umbilicus to the upper edge of the pubic bone is 5 divisions.

Effects: Pain in the whole belly like a knife turning around inside; stomach feels full and hot with pain going down to the urethra with anuria; sweating and pruritis of the scrotum; pain in the testicles; cramping in the back and in the knee; a hot feeling below the umbilicus; vaginal discharge; discharge from the urinary tract in women; pain and coldness around the umbilicus; menorrhagia; menstrual cramps; discharge and/or dizziness after confinement; itching in the vagina; feeling of gas ascending from the lower abdomen; edema; child's fontanel does not close (direct moxa here and CV-9).

Treatment: Needle: 1/2 to 3/4 inch.
Moxa: 5-100 times.

Stimulus: Down to urethra and up to the umbilicus.

13.2 **Chi Hai** *sea of chi* **CV-6**

Location: 1 and 1/2 divisions below the center of the umbilicus.

Effects: Cold feeling from below the umbilicus going up to the stomach and the heart; incessant vomiting; frightened and cannot sleep; abdomen swollen with panting; pain and cold feeling below the xiphoid process; red face; Yang Chi empty (penis is weak); weak Chi in the five viscera; true Chi deficient (lack of energy of the whole body); chronic Chi disease (gastric pain, stomachache, not enough energy when walking, etc.); body becoming emaciated; weakness in the four limbs; hernia and/or pain/inflammation in testicle; abdomen swollen like a drum; spermatorrhoea; after the "cold" flu (flu without fever), a testicle retracts into the body from cramping; feeling of coldness in four limbs; constipation; hematuria; acute angina pectoris; after intercourse during menstruation the woman becomes thinner and thinner (use needle and moxa on this point); hemorrhage of the womb; bed-wetting; red and/or white vaginal discharge; incessant discharge after confinement; irregular period; dysmenorrhea; numbness of the bladder where the patient cannot urinate; wet dreams (with excessive loss of semen); panting; asthma; any disease below the umbilicus.

Treatment: Needle: 1/2 to almost 1 inch.
Moxa: 7 to 100 times.

Stimulus: Down to the urethra and up to the umbilicus.

13.3 **Shi Men** *stone door* **CV-5**

Location: 2 divisions below the center of the umbilicus.

Effects: Abdomen swollen, painful and hot; incessant diarrhea; inflammation of the cecum; vomiting of blood; chronic indigestion in children; difficulty in urinating, with deep yellow or red colored urine; gonorrhea; cramping of scrotum such that the testicles are retracted into the body; after childbirth, incessant bleeding; hemorrhage from uterus; incessant but scanty menstruation.

Treatment: Needle: 1/2 to 1 inch.
Moxa: 7 to 27 times. **No needle or moxa on women**, stimulation of this point is reported to cause sterility.

Stimulus: Down to the urethra.

Note: According to the old book, this point is forbidden to use on women because it can cause sterility. I have used this point on seven women, including my wife, who have not wanted any more children. All of them were able to conceive after using this point. Some seemed to conceive more quickly than usual. However, you should still believe that it might cause sterility because every person is different.

13.4 **Kuan Yuan** *gate origin* **CV-4**

Location: On midline, three divisions below the center of the umbilicus.

Effects: Abdomen painful down to sexual organs; dyspnea; dysentery; cholera; diarrhea; prolapse of rectum; lines of pain around navel; abdomen swollen like a drum; fibroids below navel make an upturned cup; dysuria; hematuria; urinary incontinence; spermatorrhea; impotence; wet dreams (no moxa for this point, only needle); vaginal discharge; irregular menstruation; light menstruation for long periods; dysmenorrhea; prolapse of uterus; abdomen painful after confinement; retained placenta; leukorrhea and gonorrhea; hernia; inflammation of testicles; bed wetting in children; amenorrhea; frequency of urination at night; severe weakness of the entire body; women cannot conceive.

Treatment: Needle 3/4 to 1 inch; if treating a thin woman, use 1/2 inch.
Moxa: 7 to 100 times.
No Needle or Moxa for pregnant women.

Stimulus: Down to the urethra.

13.5 **Jung Ji** *middle extremity* **CV-3**

Location: On the midline, 4 divisions below the center of the umbilicus.

Effects: Lack of yang and weakness of the whole body; a cold feeling in abdomen with cold sensations going up to the heart; a lump below the navel (sometimes moving); spermatorrhea; dropsy; fainting without sensation; leukorrhea; dysuria; urinary incontinence; frequent micturition; hungry without appetite; irregular menstruation; dysmenorrhea; menorrhagia; excessive white or red vaginal discharge; pruritis vulvae; vaginal orifice swollen and painful; prolapse of uterus; pain in vagina; retained placenta; incessant discharge after confinement (no discharge after childbirth); impotence; spermatorrhea; hematuria; hernia; inflammation or pain in testicles; gonorrhea; leukorrhea; hemorrhage of the vagina; itching in the vagina; woman's body becoming thin after intercourse during menstruation; woman cannot conceive.

Treatment: Needle: 3/4 to 1 inch.
Moxa: Start at 5 times, stop at 100 times.

Stimulus: Down to the urethra.

13.6 **Chu Gu** *crooked bone* **CV-2**

Location: 5 divisions below the center of the umbilicus, on the upper edge of the pubic bone.

Effects: Weakness in five viscera; spermatorrhea; lower abdomen swollen or full and extremely painful; retention of urine; cystitis; red or white vaginal discharge; gonorrhea; metrorrhagia; menorrhagia, (uterus does not reduce in size within the normal period after childbirth); inflammation of the uterus; hemorrhage of the uterus.

Treatment: Needle: 1/2 inch or a little more.
Moxa: start at 7 times, stop at 100 times.

Stimulus: Goes through the entire sexual ogan and perineum.

13.7 **Hui Yin** *perineum* **CV-1**

Location: On the midline, between the sexual organ and the anus. Note: The old book says this point is between the anus and sexual organ, on the midline of the body. This looks simple but is not simple at all. In some women the vagina is close while in other women the vagina is farther from the anus. In the female (far or close) it is easy to find the location. In the male, there are no boundaries between the penis and the anus. But when the penis is stronger, one can touch the bottom of the penis and determine the distance between the penis and the anus. When the penis is soft, you cannot get the correct distance. In my experience, this point is 1/2 inch in front of the edge of the anus on the midline. Insert through the tissue connecting the anus to the scrotum. Also, the reaction goes to the penis and/or the vagina and the whole scrotum when the point is correct. To locate this point, tell the patient to lie down on one side and bend both legs high up (fetal position). The needle is inserted perpendicular to the point.

Effects: Lack of yin, with headaches; all disease of perineal area; pruritis vulvae; pain or swelling in the vagina; prolapse of the uterus; pain between the anus and sexual organ with a complete blockage of the passage of urine and faeces; penis feels cold and painful; itching in the anus (pruritis ani); chronic piles; amenorrhea in young women; burning sensation in the chest or heart; pain on the skin of whole body; constant erection (also use BL-18 and BL-23 to help this case); sudden unconsciousness from shock; drowning (insert needle 1 inch; if the patient is still alive both urine and feces will come out; if the patient is dead there will be no reaction).

Treatment: Needle: 1/2 to 3/4 inch; for drowning, 1 inch.
Moxa: 3 times.

Stimulus: Reaction through the whole sexual organ.

Note: Note: The old book says no needle, this is not true.

13.8 **Nang Di** *bottom of scrotum* **X.SC. 1**

Location: At the bottom of the scrotum, between the two testicles, on the midline. Note: the point is on the middle of the tissue line. To locate this point, let the male patient stand up and find the point. If one testicle is higher and one lower, the point is still on the tissue line.

Effects: Local hernia, and any problem of testicle and scrotum; weakness of penis; cold in the scrotum; loosening of scrotum; weak force of urination; weak force of ejaculation; sexual frigidity.

Treatment: **No Needle.**
Moxa: 7 times (size of 1/2 grain of rice).

Stimulus: Reaction to perineum.

Note: All charts which place this point posterior to the scrotum are incorrect.

13.9 **Gwie Tau** *head of penis* **XP-1**

Location: On the upper side of the penis on the center line, on the neck between the body and head.

Effects: Weakness of the penis.

Treatment: Needle: 1/16 inch.
No Moxa.

Stimulus: Local pain stimulus.

Section 14 **Lower Abdomen, Lateral Two Divisions**

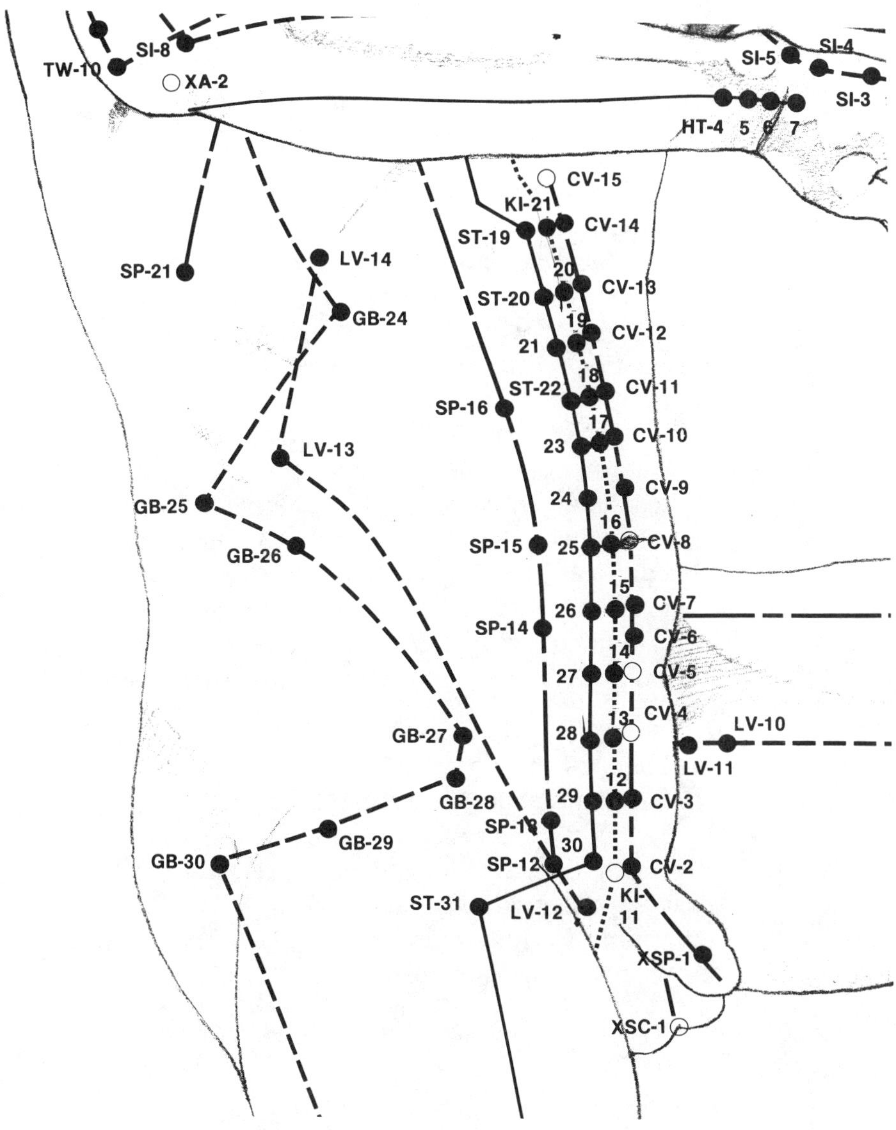

Lower Abdomen

Illustration 16

14.1 **Tien Shu** *heavenly pivot* **ST-25**

Location: Two divisions lateral from the center of the umbilicus.
Note: There are 8 divisions between the two nipples. In men or young girls, the correct measurement is easy to get. For older women it is difficult. Women's breasts are divided into three shapes: a) round and firm; b) long; c) irregular, hung to one side. For the round and long shapes, the measurement is usually easy to get. For the irregular shape it is difficult. Women who are nursing have breasts which vary in size and the measurement is also difficult. In these cases of irregularity find the edges of each breast and then the midpoints between these edges at the center of the chest; the distance between these two points should be eight divisions.

Effects: All problems with intestines; acute or chronic problems of the stomach; dysentery (white or red); cholera; full feeling in stomach with vomiting; pain in lower abdomen; diarrhea with swelling on abdomen and panting; edema of the whole body; irregular menstruation; leukorrhea; sterility; retention of urine; tapeworm; cold feeling around umbilicus, sometimes going up to the chest.

Treatment: Needle: 1/2 to 3/4 inch; **No Needle for Pregnant Women**.
Moxa: 5 to 100 times.

Stimulus: Straight down 2-3 inches from this point.

14.2 **Da Jiuh** *big great* **ST-27**

Location: Below the center of the umbilicus two divisions, and lateral two divisions (two divisions lateral to CV-5).

Effects: Swelling in the lower abdomen; frequency of thirst and difficulty in urination; hernia; pain or inflammation in the testicles; ovaritis; insomnia caused by fright; weakness of the limbs.

Treatment: Needle: 1/2 to 3/4 inch.
Moxa: 5 times.

Stimulus: Straight down to the scrotum.

14.3 **Shui Dao** *water path* **ST-28**

Location: Three divisions down from the center of the umbilicus and lateral two divisions (two divisions lateral to CV-4).

Effects: Cramping in the lumbar area of back; catarrh of the bladder; retention of urine and feces; inflammation of testicles; losing yang (see: CV-8); coldness in the vagina and uterus; irregular menstruation; amenorrhea; swelling in the lower abdomen in women; edema of whole body.

Treatment: Needle: 1/2 to 3/4 inch.
Moxa: 5 times.

Stimulus: Straight down to the sexual organ.

14.4 **Gui Lai** *coming back* **ST-29**

Location: Four divisions under umbilicus, lateral 2 divisions. Also two divisions lateral from CV-3.

Effects: Hernia; inflammation of the testicles; pain in the penis; testicles retracted into the body; inflammation of ovaries; amenorrhea; pain in the vagina; sterility; gas in the lower abdomen moving up and down. This point has a special effect on the male and female genitalia.

Treatment: Needle: 1/2 inch.
Moxa: 5 times.

Stimulus: For males, the reaction is straight down to the testicles. For females, the reaction is felt in the vagina and urethra.

14.5 **Chi Chung** *chi rushing* **ST-30**

Location: Five divisions below the umbilicus, lateral two divisions.
Note: A big pulse is close to this point (femoral artery).

Effects: Chi rushing up to the chest; swelling of the abdomen; inflammation of the testicles; testicles retract into the body; pain in the penis; sterility; inflammation of the ovaries; menorrhagia; difficulty in delivering a baby (dystocia); retained placenta; too much secretion on the part of the woman during sexual intercourse; tipped uterus; pain in the small intestine.

Treatment: Needle 1/4 to 1/2 inch.
Note: In the old book, it is forbidden to needle this point because of the large pulse close to the point. Before treating this point, find the pulse and use a fingernail to protect the pulse, then insert the needle.
Moxa: 3 to 7 times.

Stimulus: Up to LV-14, down to LV-11.

Note: All of the points between the xiphoid process and the pubic bone should be needled while the patient is lying down.

14.6 **Yin Lian** *screen of sexual organ* **LV-11**

Location: Two divisions below Chi-Chung (ST-30) in the crease between the lower abdomen and the top of the thigh, in the hollow at the upper side of the big tendon. Note: To locate this point, have the patient sit with the legs spread, find the big tendon in the crease between thigh and lower abdomen; the point is in the hollow on the upper side of the tendon.

Effects: Sterility; tipped uterus; local pain.

Treatment: Needle 1/2 to 3/4 inch.
Moxa: 3 times.

Stimulus: Up to the respective sexual organ, down to the inner side of the thigh.

Section 15 **Points in the Shoulder Area**

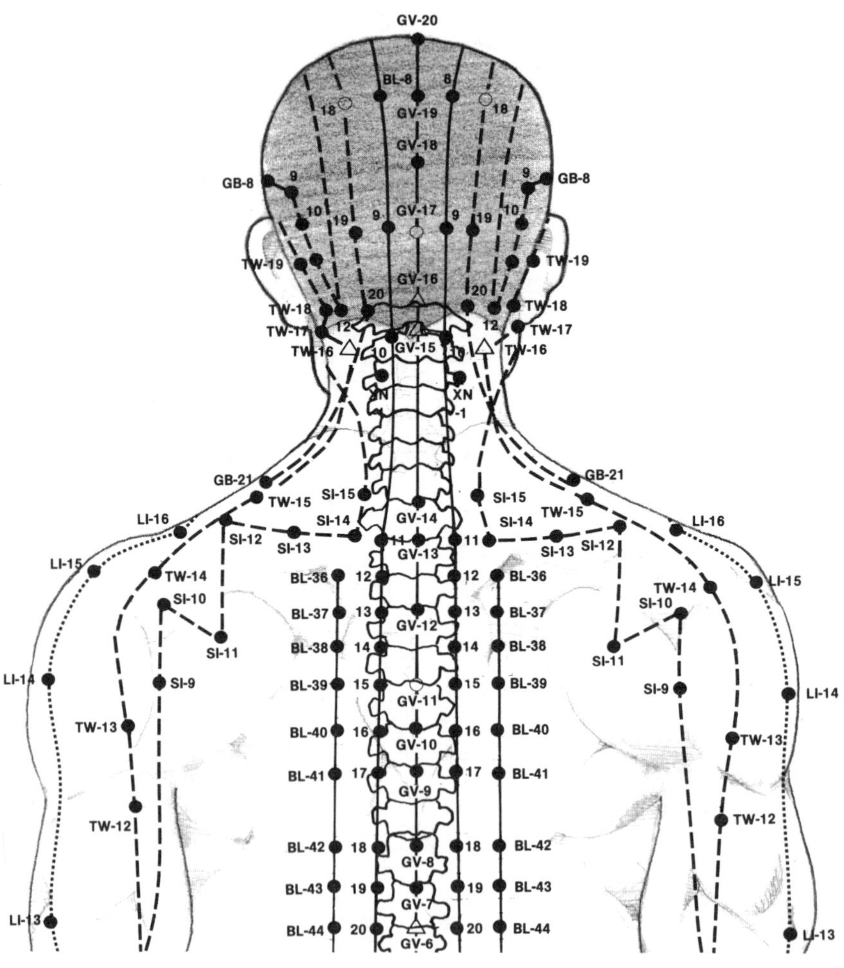

Points in the Shoulder Area
Illustration 17

15.1 **Jian Jing** *shoulder well* **GB-21**

Location: One-half way between the end of the clavicle equal with LI-16 and the base of the neck, on the top of the muscle.
Note: To locate this point, use the thumb and middle finger to hold the muscle, use the first finger to press down on the middle of the muscle until you feel the muscle divide in half. Between the two halves is the point.

Effects: Headache on the top of the head; stiffness or cramping of the neck; pain on the shoulder and arm; patient cannot raise their arm up to the head; after a stroke, difficulty in breathing wih phlegm in the mouth and cannot speak; difficult labor; premature labor or miscarriage with cold limbs; carbuncle in the breast; cancer in the breast; inflammation of the breast glands; chest feels tight; difficulty in breathing during a fever; body overheating and the chest feels painful.

Treatment: Needle: 1/2 inch and 1 and 1/2 inch.
Do not needle this point if a woman is pregnant. No deep needle on patients with a history of heart problems.
Moxa: 5 times.

Stimulus: Shallow needle: reaction up to temple and down to shoulder. Deep needle (1 and 1/2 inch): reaction down the chest to the 10th rib.

15.2 **Jian Yu** *shoulder bone* **LI-15**

Location: On the top of the humerus bone below the acromion, at the midline of the arm. Raise the arm, the two muscles will form a hollow which is the point.

Effects: Hemiplegia; pain and weakness in the shoulder and arm; patient cannot raise their arm up to the head; cannot turn head; hot feeling on four limbs; spermatorrhea after talking a long time; emaciation; scrofula; fatty tumor on the skin.

Treatment: Needle: 1/2 to 3/4 inch; needle 75 degrees up to down.
Moxa: not over 7 times; if used over 7 times it will cause atrophy of the upper arm muscle. 5 times is good.

Stimulus: Reaction down the arm half way to the elbow on the outside of the upper arm.

15.3 **Jiuh Guu** *great bone* **LI-16**

Location: Between the clavicle and scapula, on the back of the shoulder.
Note: Some charts put this point on the front side of the shoulder; this is incorrect.

Effects: Convulsions in children; vomiting blood; toothache in the teeth of the lower jaw; patient cannot raise the shoulder and arm; dyspnea.

Treatment: Needle: 1/4 to 1/2 inch.
Moxa: 7 times.

Stimulus: Reaction inside the middle of the arm half way to the elbow.

Section 16 **Midline of the Back, Governing Vessel**

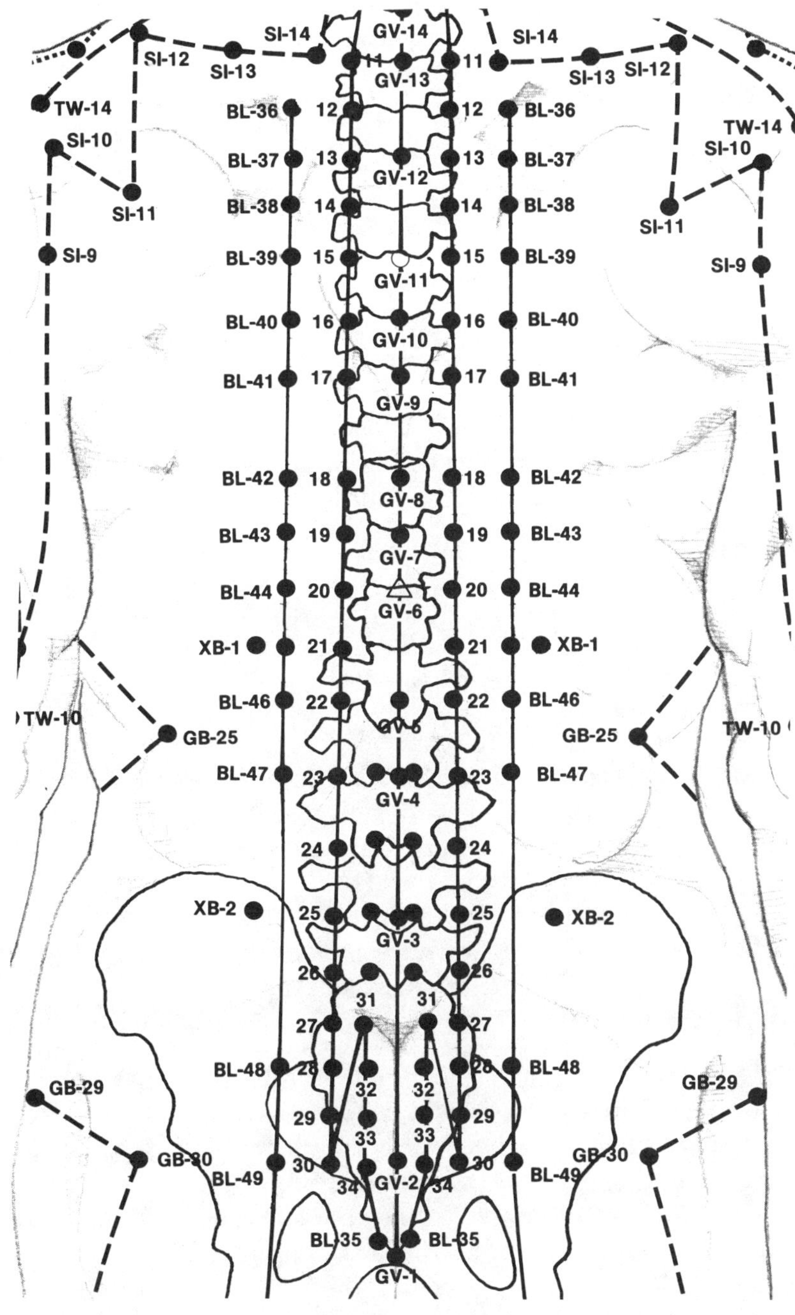

Midline of the Back

Illustration 18

Note: For all points located between two vertebrae, the pressing finger should be placed parallel to and between the two vertebrae.

16.1 **Da Chui** *big hammer* **GV-14**

Location: Between the seventh cervical and the first thoracic vertebrae.

Effects: Takes away overheating in the chest area; treats any body fever; malaria; pulmonary emphysema; tuberculosis; coughing; asthma; hysteria; flu with high temperature and cold sensations; a pressing feeling in the chest; difficulty breathing deeply and talking; cramping of the neck; vomiting; nose bleeding; cold in the four limbs.

Treatment: Needle: 1/2 inch, 1 inch; acrossing needle 1 and 1/2 inch.
Moxa: 5 times, or by the age of the patient.

Stimulus: For needle 1/2 inch deep, the stimulus goes up to the neck and down the spine. For needle 1 inch deep, the stimulus is to the chest area. For the needle inserted 1 and 1/2 inches crossing to the left, the stimulus goes up to the left side of the neck; if the needle is inserted crossing to the right, the stimulus goes up to the right side of the neck.

Note: The needle should be inserted at a 45 degree angle from GV-14 toward the left, or toward the right, until it is 1 and 1/2 inches deep.

Note: The needle must stay in the middle of the muscle tissue. To locate this point, the patient should bend their neck forward. Normally, there are three prominent vertebrae; the middle one is larger and higher than the other two and the bottom of the middle vertebra is also wider than the other two. This bone is the seventh cervical vertebra, below which is the first thoracic vertebra. The point is in between these two bones on the center line. The pressing finger should be placed between and parallel to the two vertebrae, the needle should slide in along the top of the nail. Treat this point with the patient's head bent forward. The needle should be inserted perpendicular to the skin, which will put it at an 85 degree angle, up to down, with the level of the floor.

Locating this point can be difficult if the patient does not have the three prominent vertebrae, the patient may have only two, or only one. Fat people will not have any prominent vertebrae. If you cannot correctly distinguish the first thoracic vertebrae, all the points below it on the back will be wrong. After some experience in judging this point, it will be easier to find. The old book says this point is at the height of the shoulders. For some people this is correct, but most people's shoulders slant a little downwards from the neck, and the point would then be higher than the level of the shoulders.

16.2 **Tao Dao** *pottery path* **GV-13**

Location: Between the first and second thoracic vertebrae, on the center line. To locate this point, have the patient bend the neck forward.

Effects: Malaria; tuberculosis; high fever with cold sensations (flu); cramping on the neck and shoulders.

Treatment: Needle: 1/2 inch or a little more.
Moxa: 5 times.

Stimulus: Goes down the spine. You can also stimulate this point laterally. For the acrossing needle which is inserted clearly to the side, the stimulus will go up to the neck (in the same manner as GV-14). For the acrossing needle which is inserted lower, the stimulus will go down the appropriate side of the back.

16.3 **Shen Juh** *body pillar* **GV-12**

Location: Between the third and fourth thoracic vertebrae

Effects: Furuncle; pain on the spine; tuberculosis; coughing; neurasthenia; cramping with high fever; delirium; homicidal mania; convulsions in children.

Treatment: Needle: 1/4 to 1/2 inch.
Moxa: 5 times.

Stimulus: Up and down the spine from this point.

16.4 **Shen Dao** *spirit path* **GV-11**

Location: Between the fifth and sixth thoracic vertebrae.

Effects: Cardiac diseases in general; neurasthenia; forgetfulness; slackness of the jaw; convulsions in children.

Treatment: **No Needle.**
Moxa: 5 times.

Stimulus: While applying direct moxa the reaction will be felt in the heart.

16.5 **Ling Tai** *spirit tower* **GV-10**

Location: Between the sixth and seventh thoracic vertebrae.

Effects: Dyspnea; patient cannot lie down; furuncle; overcooling; coughing.

Treatment: Needle: 1/2 inch.
Moxa: 3 times.

Stimulus: Up and down the spine from this point.

16.6 **Jyh Yang** *extreme yang* **GV-9**

Location: Between the seventh and eighth thoracic vertebrae.

Effects: Jaundice; dyspnea; difficulty speaking; loins and back painful; stomach feels cold and cannot eat; four limbs swollen; borborygmus (rumbling stomach); scrofula.

Treatment: Needle: 1/2 inch.
Moxa: 3 to 7 times.

Stimulus: Up and down the spine from this point.

16.7 **Ming Men** *gate of life* **GV-4**

Location: Between the second and the third lumbar vertebrae; also under the number fourteen vertebra.

Note: In the old book, it is taught that this point is at the same level as the umbilicus. For a small percentage of people, this is correct; for most it is incorrect. For fat people, the umbilicus is lower than this point. To find the correct point, count the vertebrae from the first thoracic vertebra to the fourteenth (lumbar 2) vertebra. From the iliac crest, directly across to the vertebra, the intervertebral space is at #16, or below the #4 lumbar vertebra. Two vertebra above this point is GV-4.

Effects: Weakness of the kidneys with lumbar ache; spermatorrhea; dizziness of the eyes; tinnitus; impotence; coldness and cramping of the four limbs; severe headache; very high temperature; dizziness of the head; skin dry with no perspiration; epilepsy in children; meningitis; convulsions; cramping; red or white vaginal discharge; menorrhagia; malaria; pain in intestines; hemorrhoids and bleeding of the rectum; diarrhea; incontinence of urine; the pupil of the eye suddenly cannot see (use moxa on this point and needle on BL-18).

Treatment: Needle: 1/2 to 1 inch.
Moxa: 3 to 30 times.
Note: Do not moxa this point on young males under 20 years of age; it will cause impotence. On males 20-25 years of age, if the body is not weak, you should not use moxa, it will cause impotence for the rest of their life.

Stimulus: For shallow needle, stimulus is down to the coccyx. For deep needle, up to one inch, the reaction is up to the umbilicus.

16.8 **Yang Guan** *gate of yang* **GV-3**

Location: Under the number sixteen vertebra between #4 and #5 lumbar vertebrae.

Effects: Lumbago; neuritis or inflammation of the knees; premature ejaculation; cannot control the urine.

Treatment: Needle: 1/2 to 1 inch.
Moxa: 5 to 100 times.

Stimulus: Down to the coccyx.

16.9 **Yao Yu** *loins yu* **GV-2**

Location: Below the #21 vertebra, and above the top of the coccyx.

Note: To locate this point, have the patient lie on one side with both legs bent close to the chest. This point is between the sacrum and the coccyx. Touch the coccyx, and move your finger up to the sacrum. You will find a cleft; the needle should be inserted through the center of the cleft.

Effects: Lumbar pain; back pain; patient cannot bend forward or backward; coldness; stiffness; numbness below the lumbar area; patient cannot sit or lie down; bed wetting in children; amenorrhea; malaria with high fever; flaming sensation in the four limbs after the flu.

Treatment: Needle: 1/2 to 3/4 inch.
Moxa: 5 times.

Stimulus: Up to the lumbar vertebrae.

16.10 **Chang Chyang** *long strong* **GV-1**

Location: 1/2 inch behind the anus on the center line. To locate this point, position the patient the same as for GV-2 (Yao-Yu).

Effects: Lumbar area stiff; patient cannot bend forward or backwards; madness; urination and defecation difficult; hemorrhage of the rectum; prolapse of the rectum; piles; inflammation of rectum; diarrhea; hernia; gonorrhea; spermatorrhea caused by fright; losing of the yang; cramping of the penis; vomiting of blood; depression of fontanel area in child; convulsions and cramping; vision abnormal.

Treatment: Needle: 1/2 to 3/4 inch.
Moxa: 5 to 30 times.

Stimulus: Runs around the whole anus; for some people this point is very painful.

Note: To locate this point, bend the leg so that the knee touches the chest, treat with the patient in this position.

Section 17 **Points Lateral To The Spine**

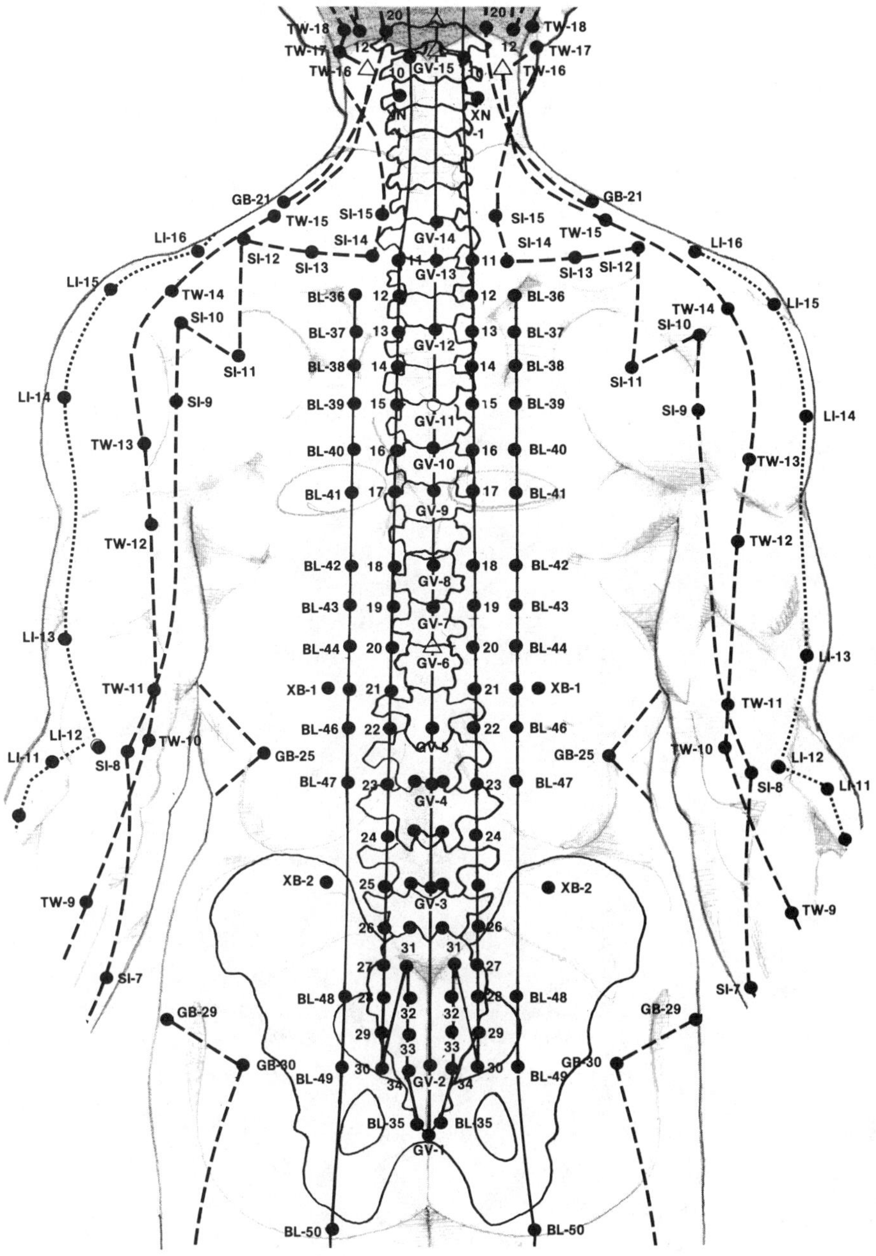

Points lateral to the spine

Illustration 19

One and One Half Divisions and Three Divisions

There are three factions of thought concerning the correct location of the bladder points on the back; one is that they lie 1 and 1/2 and 3 divisions laterally from the center of the spine; another is that they lie 2 and 4 divisions laterally from the center of the spine; the last is that the points lie 1 and 1/2 and 3 divisions from the edge of the spine. These three theories are mentioned in the old books. Most acupuncturists follow the first theory. According to my 40 years of experience, I found the first faction of thought the most correct.

The lateral divisions are measured according to the patient's finger division. Some people however have a finger division which is out of proportion to the rest of their body. This makes the measurments on the back incorrect. If the patient's finger measurement is wrong, there is a special technique for finding the correct measurement by the back muscles. Press with your thumb nail laterally from the center of the spine until you feel a natural depression in the muscles. The first depression will be 1 and 1/2 divisions from the spine, the second depression will be 3 divisions from the spine.

17.1 **Da Chu** *big shuttle* **BL-11**

Location: 1 and 1/2 divisions lateral from the intervertebral space between #1 and #2 thoracic vertebrae (across from GV-13).

Effects: With the flu, high fever without perspiration and cold sensations of the body; stiffness of the neck and coughing; headache; dizziness; dizziness of the eye; pleurisy; hot feelings in the whole chest; dysphonia; malaria; madness; arthritis of the knee;

Treatment: Needle: 1/4 to 1/2 inch (mostly 1/4 inch).
Moxa: 3 times.

Stimulus: Up to the shoulder and the neck.

Note: To locate this point, have the patient bend their head forward, find the intervertebral space under #1 thoracic vertebra, and move laterally 1 and 1/2 finger divisions from the center line of the spine.

17.2 **Feng Men** *wind gate* **BL-12**

Location: Lateral 1 and 1/2 divisions from intervetebral space between #2 and #3 thoracic vertebrae.

Effects: Takes away overheating from the lungs and body; stiffness of the neck after the flu; dyspnea; sneezing; runny nose; nose bleeding; all nose problems; pleurisy; hot feeling in the chest; bronchitis with coughing; whooping cough (pertussis); tuberculosis; vomiting; jaundice; pain in the chest and back; carbuncle on back; asthma.

Treatment: Needle: 1/4 to 1/2 inch.
Moxa: 5 times.

Stimulus: Up to the neck and the shoulders.

17.3 **Feu Yu** *lung yu* **BL-13**

Location: 1 and 1/2 divisions from the intervertebral space beween #3 and #4 thoracic vertebrae; also 1 and 1/2 divisions lateral from GV-12.

Effects: Takes away overheating in the five solid organs; tuberculosis; withering of the lungs; dyspnea; hemoptysis; coughing; shortness of breath after lying down; pneumonia; bronchitis; carditis; numbness of the heart; pruritis and pain on the skin; fatty tumor on the skin; stiffness of the neck and back; hunchback; inflammation of the mouth; dryness of the mouth and tongue; vomiting; vomiting of stomach fluid after eating; insomnia.

Treatment: Needle: 1/4 to 1/2 inch.
Moxa: 3 to 100 times.

Stimulus: Up to the shoulders and laterally a little down the back. A strong stimulus will be felt in the chest.

17.4 **Shin Yu** *heart yu* **BL-15**

Location: 1 and 1/2 divisions lateral from the intervertebral space between #5 and #6 thoracic vertebrae, also lateral from GV-11.

Effects: Takes away overheating in the five solid organs; carditis; frightened in the heart; heart palpitations; chest feels uncomfortable and sad; forgetfulness; tuberculosis; mute; madness; epilepsy; hemiplegia and cannot lie on one side; wet dreams; gonorrhea; impotence; dim vision; hemoptysis; hematemesis; epistaxis; jaundice; stenosis of the esophagus; a child who is several years old with difficulty talking (use moxa).

Treatment: Needle: 1/4 to 1/2 inch.
Moxa: 3 to 5 times.

Stimulus: Goes laterally and a little down the back.

17.5 **Ger Yu** *diaphragm yu* **BL-17**

Location: 1 and 1/2 divisions lateral from the intervertebral space between #7 and #8 thoracic vertebrae (also across from GV-9).

Effects: Carditis; cardiomegaly; numbness of the heart; pleurisy; diaphragm cramping; dyspnea; bronchitis; periostitis; catarrh in stomach; cancer of the stomach; vomiting; stenosis of the esophagus; anorexia; catarrh of the intestines; hemorrhage of intestines; tired in four limbs; excessive perspiration; night sweating; carbuncles and abcesses; itching sores; all skin diseases.

Treatment: Needle: 1/4 to 1/2 inch.
Moxa: 3 to 10 times.

Stimulus: Goes to both sides of the back.

17.6 **Gan Yu** *liver yu* **BL-18**

Location: 1 and 1/2 divisions lateral from the intervertebral space between #9 and #10 thoracic vertebrae.

Effects: Takes away overheating in the five solid organs; intercostal pain; pain of the sternum; eyes dim from overeating spicy foods; eyes weepy and dizzy; inflammation of eyeball and film over iris; pterygium; all eye disease; bad temper; jaundice; hemoptysis; hematemesis; enlargement of the liver.

Treatment: Needle: 1/2 inch.
Moxa: 3 to 7 times.

Stimulus: Laterally and a little down the back; strong stimulus will be felt in the chest.

17.7 **Dan Yu** *gallbladder yu* **BL-19**

Location: 1 and 1/2 divisions lateral from the intervertebral space between #10 and #11 thoracic vertebrae.

Effects: Intermittent fever; headache; bitter taste in mouth; dryness of tongue; tonsillitis; dry vomiting; stenosis of the esophagus; jaundice; disease of the gallbladder; pleurisy; swollen under the armpits; dryness of the skin without perspiration.

Treatment: Needle: 1/2 inch.
Moxa: 3 to 5 times.

Stimulus: Across to the sides of the back.

17.8 **Pe Yu** *spleen yu* **BL-20**

Location: 1 and 1/2 divisions lateral from the intervertebral space between #11 and #12 thoracic vertebrae (GV-6).

Effects: Takes away overheating in the five solid organs; cramping in the stomach; weakness of the stomach; anorexia; patient eats alot but remains thin; poor digestion; vomiting; undigested food in stools; catarrh in the intestines; swollen abdomen causing back pain; jaundice; edema; dyspnea; malaria.

Treatment: Needle: 1/2 to 3/4 inch.
Moxa: 3 to 7 times.

Stimulus: Laterally across the back and a little down.

17.9 **Wei Yu** *stomach yu* **BL-21**

Location: 1 and 1/2 divisions from the intervertebral space between #12 thoracic and #1 lumbar vertebrae.

Effects: Cholera; cancer in the stomach; catarrh in the stomach; cramp in the stomach; enlargement of the stomach; indigestion; borborygmus; stomachache; gastric hemorrhage; vomiting; diarrhea; abdomen swollen; gastritis; flatulence; pain on the back; hepatomegaly; jaundice; poor eyesight; night blindness of children; regurgitation of milk; green stools in children; emaciation.

Treatment: Needle: 1/2 inch.
Moxa: 3 to 10 times, or according to patient's age.

Stimulus: Laterally across the back and a little down.

17.10 **San Jiao Yu** *triple warmer yu* **BL-22**

Location: 1 and 1/2 divisions lateral from the intervertebral space between #1 and #2 lumbar vertebrae (#13 and #14 vertebrae, GV-5).

Effects: Organs congealed and swollen; abdomen and body getting thin because the patient cannot eat and drink, if they eat they vomit it back up; cramping of the stomach; anorexia; vomiting; dysentery; distended abdomen and borborygmus; stiffness of the shoulder and spine and loins, patient cannot bend backwards or forwards; headache and eyes dizzy with the flu; inflammation of the kidneys.

Treatment: Needle: 1/2 to 3/4 inch.
Moxa: 3 to 5 times.

Stimulus: Reaction felt laterally and a little down the back.

17.11 **Shen Yu** *kidney yu* **BL-23**

Location: 1 and 1/2 divisions lateral from the intervertebral space between #2 and #3 lumbar vertebrae (#14 and #15 vertebrae, GV-4).

Effects: Takes away overheating in the five solid organs; weakness of the kidneys with lumbar ache; deafness; dimness of the eyes; wet dreams; spermatorrhea; semen comes out cold; impotence; inflammation of the kidneys; edema; night urine; diabetes; gonorrhea; hematuria; lumbar area cold like ice; knees and feet cold like ice; cramping of both legs; amenorrhea; dysmenorrhea; white or red discharge; too much secretion on the part of the female during intercourse; pain in the sex organs; female emaciation after sex during menstruation; tuberculosis; weakness of the whole body; liver enlarged; headache with fever; abdomen distended; pain on both loins and lower abdomen; undigested food in stools; thirst.

Treatment: Needle: 1/2 to 3/4 inch.
Moxa: 5 to 10 times, or according to patient's age.

Stimulus: Across to the sides of the back and down a little.

17.12 **Da Chang Yu** *large intestine yu* **BL-25**

Location: 1 and 1/2 divisions lateral from the intervertebral space between #4 and #5 lumbar vertebrae (#16 and #17 vertebrae, GV-3).

Effects: Spine cannot bend; lumbar ache; borborygmus; pain around the umbilicus; diarrhea; pain in the lower belly; patient eats too much but body remains thin; catarrh in large intestine; stools contain undigested food; urination and defecation difficult; hemorrhage of the rectum; inflammation of the cecum; bed-wetting; inflammation of the kidneys; constipation.

Treatment: Needle: 1/2 to 3/4 inch.
Moxa: 3 to 5 times.

Stimulus: Laterally down the back.

17.13 **Shiao Chang Yu** *small intestine yu* **BL-27**

Location: Lateral 1 and 1/2 divisions from the intervertebral space between the 1st and 2nd sacral vertebrae.

Effects: Enteritis; dysentery with pus and blood; pain in the intestines; constipation; leukorrhea; gonorrhea; hemorrhoids; female discharge; pain on spine and sacrum; bed wetting; feet swollen; severe thirst.

Treatment: Needle: 1/2 to 3/4 inch.
Moxa: 3 to 7 times.

Stimulus: Laterally down to lower back.

17.14 **Pang Guang Yu** *bladder yu* **BL-28**

Location: 1 and 1/2 divisions lateral from the intervertebral space between #2 and #3 sacral vertebrae (#19 vertebra).

Effects: Cystitis; bed wetting; urine with yellow or red color; lumbago or pain in sacrum; dysentery; pain in the lower abdomen; inflammation of uterus (metritis); constipation; gas in abdomen, moving around; cramping in both legs and both legs without energy; abscess in area of sexual organs.

Treatment: Needle: 1/2 to 1 inch.
Moxa: 3 to 7 times.

Stimulus: Down the buttock, strongly felt down the thigh.

17.15 **Bai Huan Yu** *white circle yu* **BL-30**

Location: From the space under the last sacral vertebra (#21) and above the coccyx, lateral 1 and 1/2 divisions (lateral from GV-2).

Effects: Neuralgia or cramp in sacrum; cramp in anus; sciatica; numbness of the four limbs; constipation; metritis; anuria.

Treatment: Needle: 1/2 to 1 inch.
Moxa: 3 to 5 times.

Stimulus: Reaction is felt down to the anus, then to the sex organs, then down to the thigh.

17.16 **Shang Liao** *upper sacral foramen* **BL-31**

Location: Under the 1st sacral vertebra, (#18 vertebra), lateral 1 and 1/4 divisions.

Effects: Constipation; anuria; lower lumbar ache; sciatica; paralysis of legs; pain and cold sensations on knees; metritis; prolapse of uterus; sterility in females; menorrhalgia; inflammation of testicles; inflamed, swollen, infected ovaries.

Treatment: Needle: 1 inch.
Moxa: 5 to 7 times.

Stimulus: Radiates from the point down to the hip and outside of the thigh.

17.17 **Tsie Liao** *second sacral foramen* **BL-32**

Location: Under the second sacral vertebra (#19 vertebra) lateral 1 and 1/4 divisions.

Effects: Constipation; anuria; borborygmus; diarrhea; hematuria; gonorrhea; lower lumbar ache; sciatica; numbness from the waist down; knees with cold sensations; metritis; prolapse of the vagina; sterility in females; menorrhalgia; inflammation of testicles; the area of chest under the sternum hard and swollen.

Treatment: Needle: 1 inch.
Moxa: 5 to 7 times.

Stimulus: Laterally to both sides, and down to the buttocks.

17.18 **Jung Liao** *middle sacral foramen* **BL-33**

Location: Under the third sacral vertebra (#20 vertebra) lateral 1 division.

Effects: Constipation; urine flow irregular; diarrhea; lower lumbar ache; sciatica; metritis; menorrhalgia; sterility in females; inflammed testicles.

Treatment: Needle: 1 and 1/2 inches.
Moxa: 3 to 5 times.

Stimulus: Felt radiating to the anus, sex organ and inside the thigh.

17.19 **Hsia Liao** *lower sacral foramen* **BL-34**

Location: Under the 4th sacral vertebra (#21 vertebra) lateral 1 division.

Effects: Constipation; anuria; low back pain radiating to the testicles; borborygmus; diarrhea; intestinal hemorrhage; metritis; menorrhalgia.

Treatment: Needle: 1 and 1/2 to 2 and 1/2 inches.
Moxa: 3 to 5 times.

Stimulus: Radiates past the anus to sex organ, inner thigh and knee.

Note: To locate BL-31, BL-32,BL-33 and BL-34 have the patient sit on a stool or lie down on his side.

The above four points are referred to collectively as the "eight liao." There are some acupuncture prescriptions that include treatment of the "eight liao points." It is sometimes a little hard to locate these points. It is relatively easy to find the 18th and 21st vertebrae; and then BL-31 and BL-34. Divide the distance between BL-31 and BL-34 visually into thirds to judge the positions of BL-32 and BL-33. The sacral intervertebral depressions can usually still be distinguished. Moving laterally from the depressions you can also distinguish a small hollow at the site of the point. Needles inserted into the eight liao points should penetrate 1 inch and actually go through the sacral foramen to obtain the correct stimulus. If you cannot find the foramen initially, manipulate the needle until you get the correct stimulation.

17.20 **Hui Yang** *meeting of the yang* **BL-35**

Location: Lateral from the tip of the coccyx 1/2 division. To locate this point let the patient lie on one side of the body.

Effects: Borborygmus; diarrhea; hemorrhage of the intestines; chronic hemorrhoids; anal prolapse; sweating from genitals; pain at base of the two ischium bones.

Treatment: Needle: 1/2 inch.
Moxa: 5 times.

Stimulus: Past the anus to the bottom of the buttocks.

Section 18 **Lateral Three Divisions From Spine**

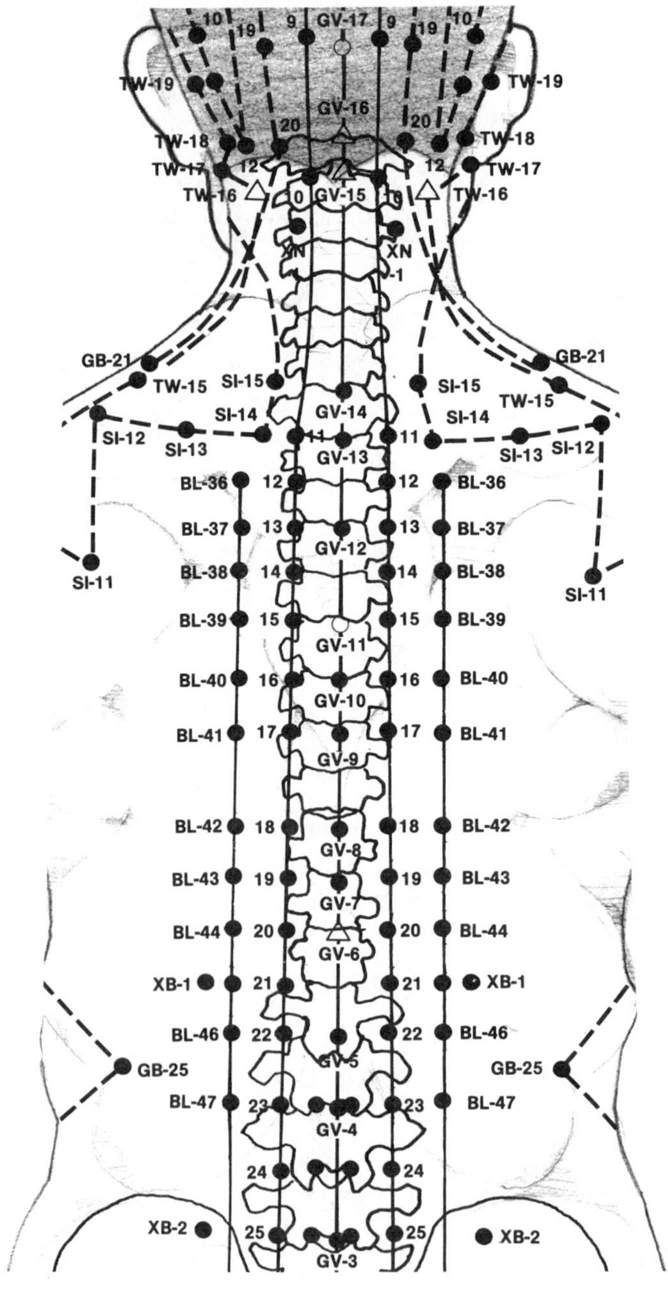

Lateral three divisions from spine

Illustration 20

18.1 **Gao Huang Yu**
area between pericardium and heart **BL-38**

Location: Between #4 and #5 thoracic vertebrae, laterally 3 divisions.

Effects: This point can cure one hundred different diseases; tuberculosis; gradual emaciation; hemoptysis; weakness of the body; dryness of the skin of the whole body; night sweating; neurasthenia; wet-dreams; spermatorrhea; forgetfulness; any weakness following recovery from a disease; hematemesis; chi running upward; malaria. During a malaria attack treat this point with the needle and the fever or chill will cease.

Treatment: Needle: 1/4 to 1/2 inch.
Moxa: 7 to 100 times.

Stimulus: Up to the neck and shoulders and arms. Strong stimulus can shake the entire shoulder.

Note: To locate this point the patient should sit straight up with their hands resting on their knees, shoulders relaxed and their head bent a little forward to prevent the scapula from covering the point. According to the old book, people under 20 should not have moxa burned on this point to help body weakness. Young bodies have more "yang;" moxa on BL-38 would stimulate overheating in the upper part of the body and therefore another disease process. When applying moxa to BL-38 one should moxa either ST-36, or CV-3, 4, or 6; so that any overheating energy will circulate through the entire body. If the patient is weak, without appetite, apply moxa to ST-36. If the patient is weak, or there is a lack of chi, or the patient has just recovered from a long period of sickness, use CV-3, 4, or 6.

18.2 **Pee Gun** *root of tumor* **XB-1**

Location: Lateral from under the #12 thoracic vertebra, 3 and 1/2 divisions.

Effects: Any tumors; cancers in the trunk; gallbladder stone or kidney stone; chronic constipation.

Treatment: **No Needle**; needle is not effective.
Use only direct moxa, the size of red bean, 14 times. If the case is severe or chronic use yellow bean size. If the tumor is on the left side, use the point on the left; if the tumor is on the right side, use the point on the right; if the tumor is in the center or on both sides of the body, moxa the point on both sides. This point is also for constipation.

Stimulus: After burning 10 direct moxa, the stimulus will be felt to front of the body.

Note: If this point needs to be treated more than once wait fourteen days between treatments.

18.3 **Tzee Shih** *palace of semen* **BL-47**

Location: Under the second lumbar vertebrae, (#14 vertebrae), and lateral 3 divisions; also lateral 1 and 1/2 divisions from BL-23.

Effects: Wet dreams; spermatorrhea; speed of urine flow irregular; pain in the sex organs; swollen sex organs; abscess in sex organ area; inflamation of the kidney; stiffness of the back; patient cannot bend forwards or backwards; indigestion; abdominal cramps; loin pain; cholera with vomiting and diarrhea.

Treatment: Needle: 1/4 to 1/2 inch.
Moxa: 3 to 7 times.

Stimulus: Stimulus to both sides, felt strongly in the front of the body.

18.4 **Yao Yen** *eye of lumbar* **XB-2**

Location: Under the fourth lumbar vertebrae (#16 vertebrae) lateral 3 and 4/5 divisions.

Effects: Tuberculosis; emaciation; body weakness; lumbar ache; red or white discharge (female); hemorrhoids with ulcers.

Treatment: Needle: 1/2 to 3/4 inch.
Moxa: 11 times each treatment.

Stimulus: Reaction down to the buttocks and hips.

Section 19 **Points on the Arms and Hands**

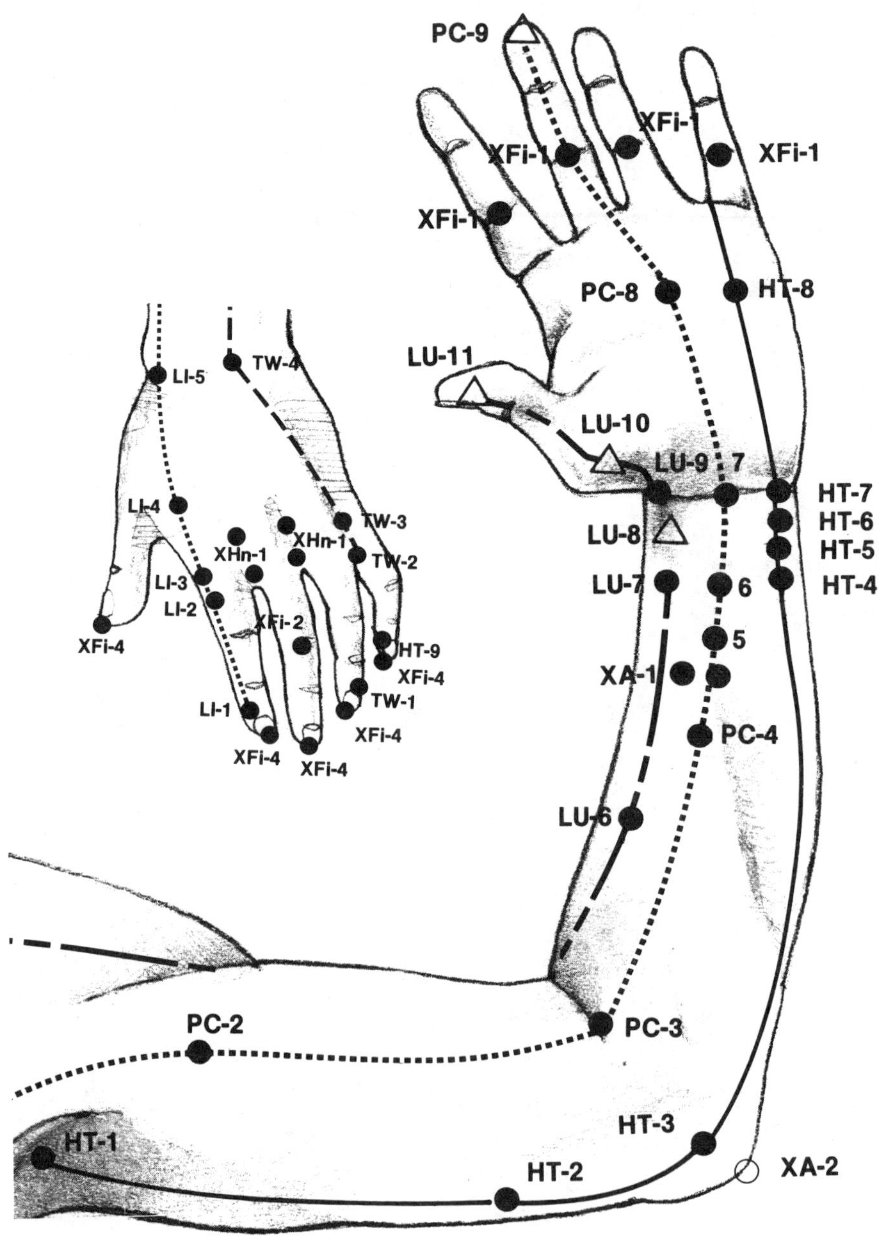

Points on the Arms and Hands

Illustration 21

19.1 **Chih Tzer** *foot marsh* **LU-5**

Location: At the crease of the elbow, on the lateral border of the tendon, between the tendon and the muscle. Bend the elbow and the point will be in the large hollow.

Effects: Tuberculosis; fever (starting in the afternoon); coughing; dyspnea (difficult breathing); emphysema; uncomfortable feelings in the heart; shortness of breath; thick phlegm in the chest; sneezing; numbness in the throat; pain on the shoulder and arm; difficulty in raising the arm; cramping of the elbow; hemoptysis; hematemesis; cramping in children; apolexy with perspiration; pain on the spine; pleurisy; malaria; the patient cries easily.

Treatment: Needle: 1/4 to 1/2 inch.
No Moxa.

Stimulus: Light electric stimulus to the hand.

Note: To treat this point the elbow should be bent slightly.

19.2 **Lieh Ch'ueh** *broken line* **LU-7**

Location: Behind the palm 1 and 1/2 divisions up from the crease of the wrist at the inner edge of the radial bone.

Effects: Facial paralysis; hemiplegia; patient cannot open the mouth to talk; laughing; tuberculosis; dyspnea; coughing; alot of phlegm in the chest; delirium; forgetfulness; migraine headache; pain on neck; scrofula; convulsions in children; melancholy feeling in the lower part of the chest; numbness in the throat; vomiting with bubbling saliva; blood and semen in urine; burning sensation while urinating; pain in the penis; weakness in the elbow or wrist; sudden swelling of the four limbs (marie's disease); cold sensation on the arms, shoulders, chest or back; fainting. This point can help move the Chi in the whole body.

Treatment: Needle: 1/4 inch.
Moxa: 3-7 times (there is a pulse here).

Stimulus: Reaction to the thumb and first finger.

Note: To locate this point, let the patient rest their arm on one side with the thumb pointing up. Use your pressing finger to protect the pulse. Put the pointing finger nail between the radius bone and pulse and place the needle on the upper side of the nail.

Note: Other factions of acupuncturists locate this point on the top of the radius bone. But this point belongs to the Lung line, a yin line, and the top of the radius bone is a yang area, thus not the proper location.

19.3 **Jing Chyu** *meridian gutter* **LU-8**

Location: In front of LU-7, one division; below the radial eminence, 1/2 division proximal to the wrist crease.

Effects: The flu with a higher fever without perspiration; malaria; coughing with the feeling that the energy is rising to the top of the body; stiffness on the chest or back; cardiac pain; emphysema and numbness in the chest; vomiting; spasm of esophagus; tonsillitis; epistaxis; hot sensations on the palm.

Treatment: Needle: a little less than 1/4 inch.
No Moxa. There is a pulse at this point.

Stimulus: Reaction down to the thumb.

Note: To locate and treat this point while protecting the pulse see the preceeding discussion of LU-7.

19.4 **Tai Yuan** *bigger abyss* **LU-9**

Location: In the hollow at the flexure of the wrist, between the radial bone and metacarpals, 1/2 division in front of LU-8.

Effects: Coughing; numbness of the chest; enlargement of the lungs; hematemesis; hemoptysis; dryness in the throat; belching; stenosis of the esophagus; pain from the chest up to the clavicle; pain in the wrist joint; hot sensation on the palms; pain on the lateral side of the arms and elbows; pain on the shoulder and back; insomnia; "crazy talking;" cold; (overcooling) panting; cardiac pain; blood in the urine; colitis.

Treatment: Needle: a little less than 1/4 inch.
Moxa: 3 times. There is a pulse at this point.

Stimulus: Reaction deep and around the wrist joint.

Note: To locate this point find the pulse and use the pressing finger nail to protect the pulse and then penetrate the point.

19.5 **Shao Shang** *young merchant* **LU-11**

Location: On the inner side of the thumb. With the palms down, the side of the hand closer to the body is the "inner" side. The side moving out away from the body is the "outer" side. With the palms up, the side closer to the body is also called the "inner" side. This is the Chinese habit, most books and charts in the west mislocate this point by mistranslating the Chinese idea of "inner." LU-11 is behind the edge of the cuticle 1/10th of an inch and directly behind the inner edge of the nail.

Effects: Throat and jaw swollen; wheezing in the throat; hemorrhage of the mouth; soft tumor under the tongue; swelling of the tongue; double tongue; decay of the tongue with parched lips; epistaxis (direct moxa); melancholy feeling in the lower part of the chest; swelling under the chest; coughing; belching; overfull feeling in the stomach; hot sensations on the palms; pain on the five fingers; thirst; patients who drink too much water and cannot eat; malaria; cerebral congestion; meningitis. Bleeding this point can take away overheating in the five solid organs. At the beginning of a stroke with the patient fainting, lockjaw, saliva running from the mouth, use the prismatic needle on this point to revive the patient.

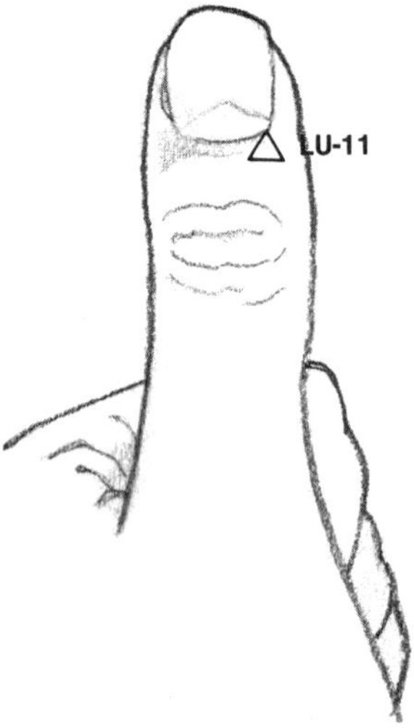

LU-11

Treatment: Needle: 1/16 inch.
No Moxa. Use moxa only for acute epistaxis, 1 to 3 times, rice grain size.

Stimulus: Severe local pain. There will be a stimulus up to the arm if the body is strong.

There is another faction of Acupuncturists who locate LU-11 on the opposite corner of the thumb. This is not correct. When locating and treating this point hold the bottom of the thumb securely so that the patient cannot move his hand.

Pericardium Line

19.6 **Chu Tzer** *crooked marsh* **PC-3**

Location: On the elbow crease on the inner side of the tendon, in the hollow between the tendon and the muscle.

Effects: Angina pectoris; patient is easily frightened; the body is hot and the patient is thirsty; patient with a dry mouth and chi moving up; hemoptysis; cholera; vomiting; pain on the elbow, the patient cannot bend or straighten it; shaking of the arm and elbow; numbness from the elbow crease to the hand.

Treatment: Needle: 1/4 to 1/2 inch.
Moxa: 3 to 5 times.
There is a pulse at this point.

Stimulus: Reaction down to the five fingers with an electric feeling.

Note: To locate this point bend the elbow a little bit and find the hollow between the muscle and the tendon. Before treating locate the pulse.

19.7 **Hsih Men** *door of the wall hole* **PC-4**

Location: On the palm side, from the wrist crease between the two tendons, up five divisions toward the elbow crease.

Effects: Angina pectoris; vomiting blood; belching; epistaxis; piles; fear of people; spirit and chi insufficient.

Treatment: Needle: 1/4 to 1/2 inch.
Moxa: 5 times.

Stimulus: Reaction up to the elbow, down to the palm.

Note: To locate this point lay the forearm on the table. Insert the needle at a 75 degree angle from the vertical axis.

19.8 **Erh Bai** *double white* **XA-1**

Location: Four divisions up from the wrist crease on the palm side of the forearm, one point is between the two tendons, the other point is on the lateral side of the lateral tendon.

Effects: Piles; prolapse of the anus; inflammation of the cecum.

Treatment: Needle: 1/4 to 1/2 inch.
Moxa: 5 times.

Stimulus: Up to the elbow, down to the fingers.

19.9 **Jian Shih** *intermediary messenger* **PC-5**

Location: Up three divisions from the palm side of the wrist crease, between the two tendons.

Effects: After the flu, chest feels hot; carditis; cardiac pain; no palpable pulse; four limbs cold; weakness of the heart; heart palpitations; stroke with phlegm coming from the mouth; dyspnea and difficulty talking; epilepsy; delirium; sudden madness; suddenly crazy (like a ghost possessed the body); frightened; cholera; dry vomiting; morning sickness; immediate vomiting after eating; vomiting with bubbly saliva; sensation of something caught in the throat; swollen under the armpits; swollen elbow; cramping of the elbow; hot sensations on the palms; menorrhalgia with a big clot in the uterus; metritis; cramping in child; crying at night; malaria; seasickness and carsickness (moxa).

Treatment: Needle: 1/4 to 1/2 inch.
Moxa: 3,5,7 or 14 times.

Stimulus: Reaction up to the elbow, down to the fingers.

19.10 **Ney Guan** *inner gate* **PC-6**

Location: On the palm side of the wrist, up two divisions from the wrist crease, between the two tendons.

Effects: All kinds of stomach diseases; angina pectoris; pericarditis; all problems of the chest and upper abdomen; stenosis of esophagus; jaundice; inflammation of the eyeball; cramping of the elbow; pain on the yin side of the arm; retained placenta; too much bleeding after labor, with dizziness.

Treatment: Needle: 1/4 to 1/2 inch.
Moxa: 3 to 5 times.

Stimulus: Reaction down to the fingers, up to the elbow. The strongest reaction will be felt in the chest.

19.11 **Da Ling** *big mound* **PC-7**

Location: Below the palm, on the crease of the wrist between the two tendons. There can be two to three wrist creases. To locate the point exactly, slide your finger nail between the two tendons up to the palm until it hits the edge of a bone. Just before the edge of the bone is the point.

Effects: High fever without perspiration and with headaches; angina pectoris; worrying in the heart; heart suspended as though hungry; epilepsy; mad speech and patient unhappy; patient always crying and frightened; incessant laughter; numbness in the throat; halitosis; dryness in the mouth; hemoptysis; hematuria; loins and chest painful; swelling under the armpits; cramping and pain on the elbow; hot sensations on palm; all fingers numb and cramped; four limbs tired; carbuncle; ringworm itching; scabies.

Treatment: Needle: 1/8 to 1/2 inch.
Moxa: 3 times.

Stimulus: Reaction down to the fingers with electric sensations.

19.12 **Lao Gung** *labor palace* **PC-8**

Location: Refer to the posterior surface of the hand, between the middle and ring finger knuckles, 1/2 division down the hand; the point is exactly opposite on the palm.

Effects: Hypertension; arteriosclerosis; after a stroke when the patient is either very angry or laughing incessantly; epilepsy; high fever for several days without perspiration; full feeling on the chest and loins; body cannot turn; chi moving up; belching; patient feels thirsty but cannot eat or drink; halitosis; mouth abscess; gingivitis in children; hematuria and blood in feces; burning piles; jaundice; hot sensations and itching skin disease on the palms.

Treatment: Needle: 1/4 inch.
Moxa: 3 times.

Stimulus: Reaction down to the middle and ring fingers.

Note: **Do not stimulate this point with the needle more than twice**, it will cause the heart to be weakened.

Note: The old book says that if the patient has nasal polyps do not moxa this point, it will make them larger.

Note: To treat this point, rest the hand flat on the table. The Acupuncturist should use the thumb as the pressing finger with heavy pressure. To insert the needle, use quick insertion to lessen the pain caused by needling this point.

19.13 **Jung Chung** *middle rushing* **PC-9**

Location: In the middle on the top of the middle finger, about 1/8 inch from the edge of the fingernail.

Effects: High temperature without perspiration; severe headache; head wants to explode; high temperature with burning sensation; angina pectoris; inflammation of the pericardium; cramping of the tongue; tongue swollen; children crying at night; hypertension; cerebral congestion; lockjaw. During the beginning of a stroke when the patient is unconscious and phlegm comes out of the mouth, use the common needle to bleed here to wake the patient up.

Treatment: Needle: 1/8 inch.
No Moxa.

Stimulus: Local pain stimulus.

Note: Hold the body of the finger, do not let the patient move. Bleed all the dark blood until fresh blood comes out.

Heart Meridian

19.14 **Shaw Hai** *young sea* **HT-3**

Location: With the arm bent at a 90 degree angle, the forearm on the vertical axis, the point is on the inner side of the elbow halfway between the tip of the humerus and the end of the ulna, one half divison up toward the hand. Use your finger to press on this point and the reaction will go up to the small finger.

Effects: Cardiac pain; Parkinson's disease; shaking of the hand; forgetfulness; headaches; neuralgia of the face; stiffness of the neck; belching.

Treatment: Needle: 1/8 to 1/4 inch.
Moxa: 3 to 7 times.

Stimulus: Strong electric stimulus to the small finger.

Note: To locate and treat this point the arm should be bent at a 90 degree angle vertically. When moxa is burnt at this point the patient should have something to prop their elbow on or hold on to in order to maintain the correct position while the moxa is burning.

Note: The following four heart points are located on the pericardium meridian side of the tendon which is found on the yin inner side of the forearm.

19.15 **Ling Dao** *soul path* **HT-4**

Location: On the inner side of the arm, 1 and 1/2 divisions proximal from the wrist crease.

Effects: Angina pectoris; sudden muteness; dry vomiting; cramping of the arm; cramping of the body.

Treatment: Needle: 1/8 to 1/4 inch.
Moxa: 3 times.

Stimulus: Up and down the heart line two to three inches. The strongest reaction will be down to the fingers or up to the elbow.

Note: To locate this point, use the pressing fingernail, touch the edge of the tendon; the needle is inserted in between the fingernail and the tendon.

19.16 **Tung Lie** *through a mile* **HT-5**

Location: One half division distal to HT-4.

Effects: Menorrhalgia; menorrhea; bed-wetting; headaches; dizziness; dizziness in the eyes; pain in the eyes; palpitations; sudden muteness; tonsillitis; face hot without perspiration; pain on the arm and elbow.

Treatment: Needle: 1/8 to 1/4 inch.
Moxa: 3 to 7 times.

Stimulus: Reaction to small finger.

19.17 **Yin Hsi** *wallhole of the yin* **HT-6**

Location: One-half division distal to HT-5.

Effects: Angina pectoris; palpitations; headaches; dizziness; cold sensations of the whole body; sudden muteness; tonsillitis; epistaxis; hematemesis; night-sweating; excessive perspiration; cholera.

Treatment: Needle: 1/8 to 1/4 inch.
Moxa: 3 to 7 times.

Stimulus: Reaction down to the small finger.

19.18 **Shen Men** *spirit door* **HT-7**

Location: On the wrist crease, at the edge of the wrist bone.

Effects: Epilepsy; foolishness; forgetfulness; patient with a red face and excessive laughter; excessive laughter; excessive crying; frightened; palpitations; melancholy feeling in the chest; angina pectoris; cardiomegaly; lack of spirit; sudden muteness; insomnia; jaundice; tonsillitis; stuffed nose; epistaxis; hemoptysis; bed-wetting; metritis; excessive bleeding after confinement (with dizziness).

Treatment: Needle: 1/4 inch.
Moxa: 3 to 7 times.

Stimulus: Strong electric stimulus down to the small finger.

Note: Heart points 4 to 7 are all on the pericardium line side of the tendon. However, HT-7 is needled at the edge of the wrist bone rather than at the edge of the tendon and is a little closer to the pericadium line relative to the other three heart points. To locate this point, use the pressing fingernail, press from HT-4 along the edge of the tendon to the edge of the wrist bone; right before the bone is the point.

19.19 **Shaw Fu** *yang mansion* **HT-8**

Location: Between the ring and small finger knuckles, proximal one-half division, on the opposite side of the hand (i.e. on the palm).

Effects: Loosening of one testicle; prolapse of the uterus; itching in the vagina; dysuria; urinary incontinence; sighing; fear of people; painful chest; sore arms; cramp in the elbow; arm and hand tired; hard to straighten hand; hot sensations on the palm; chronic malaria; chronic indigestion in children; anorexia in children. For children with chronic indigestion, there will be some yellow, glue-like fluid in this point. Insert a prismatic needle here to a depth of 1/8 inch and squeeze out the yellow, glue-like fluid until the fluid is clear.

Treatment: Needle: 1/8 to 1/4 inch.
Moxa: 3 to 7 times.

Stimulus: Strong electric stimulus to the little finger.

19.20 **Shaw Chung** *lesser rushing* **HT-9**

Location: The lower inner corner of the small fingernail.

Effects: High temperature with a full feeling in the chest; chi rushing up; dryness in the throat and mouth; eyes yellow; angina pectoris; crying; frightened conditions; heart palpitations; pain on the inner side of arm; elbow pain; difficult to straighten elbow. As a special treatment for vaginal odors use this point in conjunction with LV-2. Treat LV-2 first and then treat this point. For patient with stroke, phlegm in the mouth, fainting unconscious, and lockjaw, use the prismatic needle at this point to revive the patient.

Treatment: Needle: 1/16 inch.
Moxa: 3 times.

Stimulus: Severe local pain.

Note: To treat this point, hold the body of the little finger.

19.21 **Sze Fung** *four sewing* **XFi-1**

Location: Includes four locations: on the center of the middle crease of the four fingers (palm side).

Effects: These four points are specifically for anorexic children with chronic indigestion.

Treatment: With the prismatic needle insert to a depth of 1/16 inch, squeeze out the yellow glue-like fluid until it is clear. If the condition is very chronic or severe, treat these points 2 to 3 days in a row. Always squeeze until the yellow glue is gone; then the child should have a good appetite.

Stimulus: Local, slight pain stimulus.

Section 20 **Large Intestine Meridian**

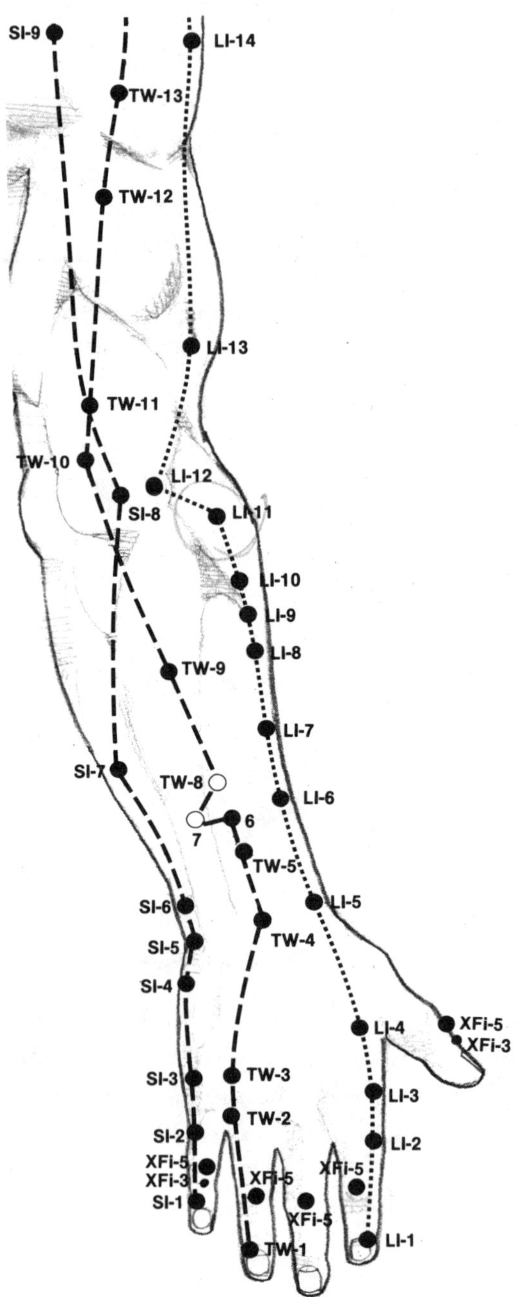

Large Intestine Meridian
Illustration 22

20.1 **Shang Yang** *merchant yang* **LI-1**

Location: On the pointing finger at the inner corner of the fingernail.

Effects: Flu with higher fever and no perspiration; cerebral congestion; swollen jaw; tonsillitis; dryness in mouth; toothaches; coughing and full a feeling in the chest; deafness; tinnitus; cataracts; leg and arm cramps; shoulder and neck stiffness; pain behind the clavicle. For patient with stroke, unconsciousness, lockjaw, use the prismatic needle to bleed this point and revive the patient.

Treatment: Needle: 1/16 inch.
Moxa: 3 times.

Stimulus: Severe local pain.

Note: To treat Shang Yang, hold the body of the finger.

20.2 **Ho Ku** *union of the valleys* **LI-4**

Location: The highest point on the muscle of the hand between the thumb and the first finger when the thumb and first finger are pressed together.

Effects: The flu with excessive thirst; high temperature without perspiration and with cold sensations; headache; stiffness of the spine; intermittent fevers and chills; migraine; swollen face; cannot close lips; muteness; mouth cannot open; toothaches; numbness in the throat; tonsillitis; dim vision; film on iris; deafness; inflammation of the otitis media; stuffed nose; every kind of mouth and face problem; itching; epistaxis; urticaria; fingers difficult to bend and straighten. After confinement, no palpable pulse, use with KI-7 and PC-5 to revive the pulse.

Treatment: Needle: 1/4 to 1/2 inch. **No Needle** for pregnant women.
Moxa: 3 to 5 times.
This point is near a pulse; touch the pulse before inserting needle.

Stimulus: Down to the thumb and pointing finger. Strongest reaction is up the arm to the top of the head.

Note: To locate this point, rest the side of the hand on the table, let the patient press the thumb and pointing finger together. Estimate the highest point on the muscle, locate the pulse and then insert the needle. However, during the treatment the thumb and the pointing finger should be loose.

Note: Some acupuncturists describe different location for this point:
1) At the corner where the first and second metacarpal bones meet.
2) When the thumb and pointing finger are pressed together, the point is at the end of the crease. These locations are incorrect.

20.3 **Yang Hsi** *yang stream* **LI-5**

Location: On the wrist crease, at the end of the first metacarpal bone, in the hollow between the two tendons. When the thumb is pointing up you can see the hollow at this area.

Effects: Crazy speech; laughter; patient visited by spectres; high temperature with melancholia in the heart; chest full with dyspnea; malaria; overcooling, coughing and vomiting of saliva; headache; conjunctivitis with a film over the iris; deafness; tinnitus; cramping of the elbow; itching; poisonous snake bites (burn three moxa here to protect the brain).

Treatment: Needle: 1/4 inch.
Moxa: 3 times.
There is a big pulse here, protect it before treating this point.

Stimulus: Reaction is deep into the wrist, out to the thumb.

20.4 **(Shou) San Li** *arm three miles* **LI-10**

Location: Two divisions below LI-11. Two divisions below the outer elbow crease on top of the muscle. Using your finger to press on this point, the muscle will divide in half; make sure you understand the correct position of LI-11 in order to determine the location of this point.

Effects: After a stroke, the arm is paralyzed; face paralyzed; cramping of the arm, difficult to straighten; numbness of arm; pain on the shoulder and back; gradual emaciation; body weakness with tuberculosis; scrofula; cholera; bowel incontinence; swollen jaw; toothache; carbuncle on breast.

Treatment: Needle: 1/4 to 1/2 inch.
Moxa: 5 times.

Stimulus: Goes down to the five fingers.

Note: To locate and treat this point, bend the arm so that the hand is flat on the chest, locate LI-11 first, then find the point on the high part of the muscle.

20.5 **Chu Chih** *crooked pond* **LI-11**

Location: At the outer crease between the humerus and radius. Bend the arm resting the hand flat on the center of the chest; at the highest part of the muscle is the point. If the patient is very thin, you cannot see this muscle; then the point will be found one division up toward the elbow crease from the meeting of the two bones.

Effects: Hemiplegia following a stroke; pain on the shoulders; pain on the upper arm; pain on the elbow; weakness of the arm; cramping of the elbow; inflammation of the elbow; melancholia and a full feeling in chest; numbness in the throat; difficulty speaking; madness with cramping; high temperature; scrofula; itching; scabies; itching eruptions on the skin; acne; whole body itching; dryness of skin; dropping off of pieces of the skin with abscesses forming on the skin; all skin diseases.

Treatment: Needle: 1/2 to 3/4 inch.
Moxa: 3, 5, or 7 or daily 7 times for a total of 200 times.

Stimulus: Usually local muscle stimulus; strong stimlus is down to the fingers, up to the shoulder.

Note: For deep elbow pain, insert the needle to a depth of 1 and 1/2 inches; for chronic skin disease, use direct moxa.

Note: To locate this point, bend the elbow and lay the hand flat on the chest. If the arm is straight, the point will be concealed.

20.6 **Wu Li** *five miles* **LI-13**

Location: On the outside center line of the upper arm, three divisions up from the elbow crease.

Effects: Pneumonia; full feeling under the chest; hemoptysis; coughing; pain on arm and elbow; cannot move the four limbs; scrofula; excessive sleeping; dimness of the eyes; malaria.

Treatment: Needle: 1/4 inch or a little deeper.
Moxa: 3 to 10 times.

Stimulus: Goes down to five fingers.

20.7 **Bei Nau** *forearm* **LI-14**

Location: On the outside center line of the arm, three divisions down from LI-15.

Effects: Arm pain, cannot raise arm; stiffness or cramping of the neck; scrofula.

Treatment: Needle: 1/4 to 1/2 inch.
Moxa: 3 to 7 times or 7 times daily to 200 times total.

Stimulus: Little down to elbow, a little up to shoulder.

Section 21 **Triple Warmer Meridian**

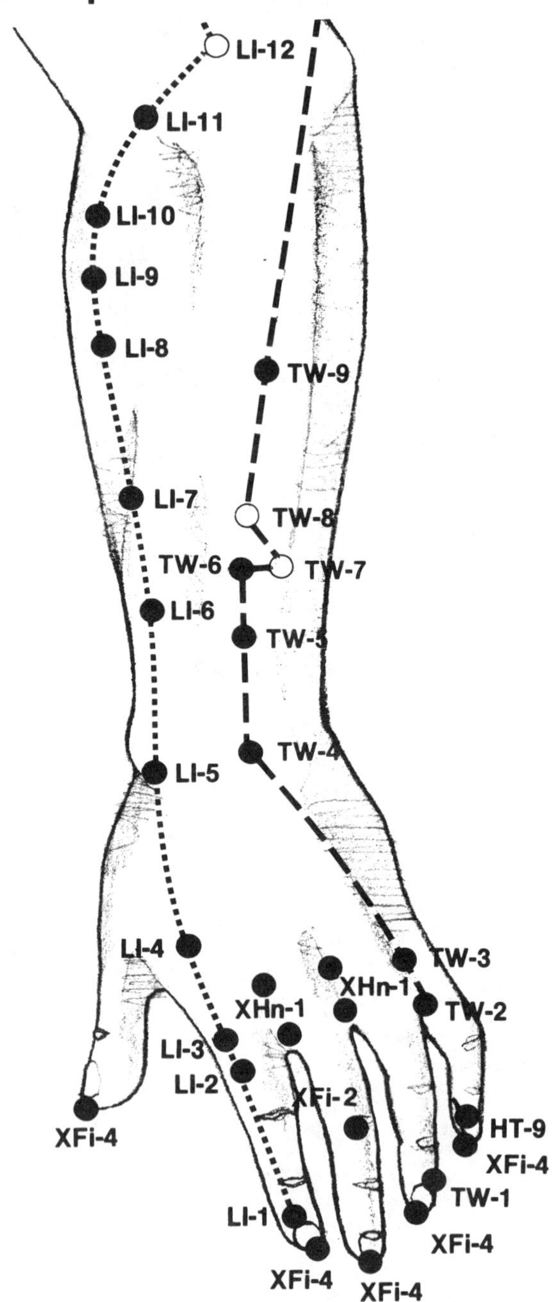

Triple Warmer Meridian
Illustration 23

21.1 **Kuan Chung** *gate rushing* **TW-1**

Location: On the outer corner of the ring finger, behind the fingernail.

Effects: High fever without perspiration; headache; cholera; belching without appetite; pain on the arm and elbow with difficulty in raising the arm; film over the iris. Bleed this point in combination with LU-11 for the following conditions: numbness of the throat; closing of the throat; tongue curled up; erosion on the surface of the tongue; small ulcers at the outer corners of the mouth; parched lips. When the patient is unconscious from a stroke, with phlegm coming from the mouth and lockjaw, use a prismatic needle to bleed this point to revive the patient.

Treatment: Needle: 1/16 inch.
Moxa: 3 times.

Stimulus: Strong, local, painful stimulus.

21.2 **Yih Men** *fluid door* **TW-2**

Location: In the web between the ring and little finger. About 1/2 division in front of the first knuckle (distal to the first knuckle).

Effects: Cramping of the elbow and arm; cannot raise arm; headache; malaria; eye is red and feels rough; acute deafness; pain in the gums; external swelling of the throat.

Treatment: Needle: 1/4 inch.
Moxa: 3 times.

Stimulus: Down the ring and small fingers.

Note: To locate this point, have the patient bend the fingers and insert the needle perpendicular to the point.

21.3 **Jung Juu** *middle islet* **TW-3**

Location: Between the fourth and fifth metacarpal bones, behind the knuckle 1/2 division (proximal to the knuckle).

Effects: High temperature without perspiration; headache; dizziness in the eyes; deafness; swelling in the throat; film over the eyes; malaria; pain on the arm and elbow; difficulty in bending or moving the five fingers.

Treatment: Needle: 1/4 inch.
Moxa: 3 times.

Stimulus: Up the wrist and down the ring finger and small fingers.

Note: To locate this point, have the patient loosely close the hand; the angle of insertion will be 80 degrees towards the wrist.

21.4 **Yang Chih** *yang pond* **TW-4**

Location: On the back of the hand, at the middle of the wrist. Relax the hand, the point is in the large hollow.

Effects: Thirst; dryness in the mouth; uncomfortable sensations in the chest; malaria; weakness or pain in the wrist; pain in the shoulder and arm, cannot raise arm.

Treatment: Needle: 1/4 inch.
Moxa: 3 to 5 times.

Stimulus: Reaction down the middle, ring and small fingers, and inside the wrist.

Note: To locate this point, lay the opened hand palm side down on the table, tell the patient to relax the hand, then find the middle hollow.

21.5 **Wai Guan** *outer door* **TW-5**

Location: On the back of the hand, 2 divisions proximal to the wrist, 2 divisions proximal to Yang Chih (TW-4); between the radial and ulnar bones.

Effects: Deafness; cramping of the arm and elbow; weakness of the arm and elbow; pain on the five fingers and weakness in the hand (use with LU-11).

Treatment: Needle: 1/4 inch or a little more.
Moxa: 3 times.

Stimulus: Reaction down the five fingers.

21.6 **Chih Kou** *branch ditch* **TW-6**

Location: On the back of the hand 3 divisions from TW-4, between the two bones.

Effects: High fever without perspiration; cholera with vomiting; patient cannot open his mouth; acute muteness; uncomfortable feeling in the chest; acute angina pectoris; a tight sensation in the chest during the "flu;" excessive blood after confinement and the patient is unconscious; chronic constipation; intercostal neuralgia; abscess in the web of the fingers; itching; ringworm; scabies.

Treatment: Needle: 1/4 to 1/2 inch.
Moxa: 3 to 14 times.

Stimulus: Reaction down to the five fingers.

Section 22 **Small Intestine Meridian**

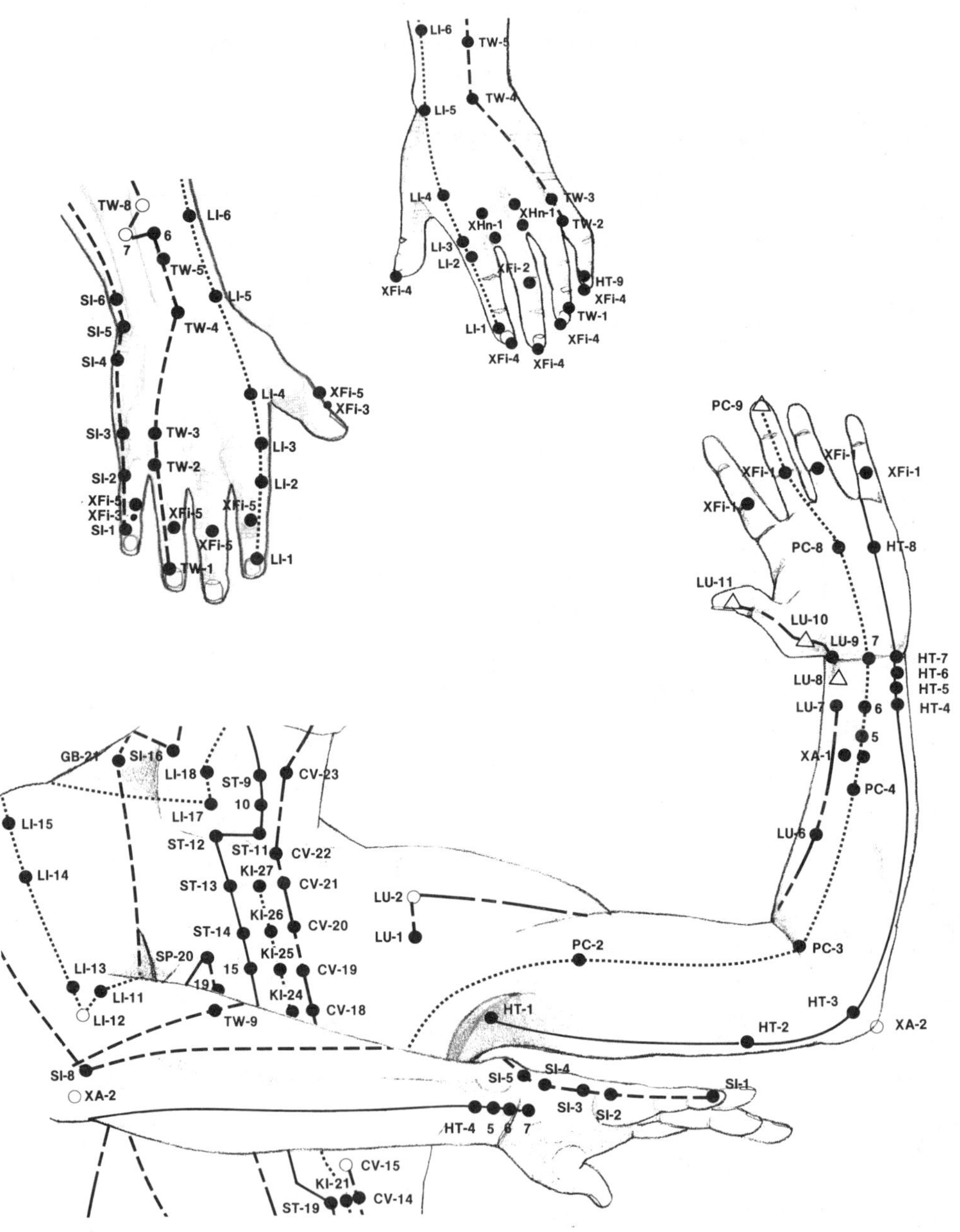

Small Intestine Meridian

Illustration 24

22.1 **Shao Tzer** *young marsh* **SI-1**

Location: Outer corner of little finger fingernail.

Effects: Malaria with cold feeling; high fever and no sweating; headache; numbness of the throat; stiffness of tongue; dryness in the mouth; melancholia of chest; frequent spitting; coughing; cardiomegaly; stiffness of neck, cannot turn the head; pain on arms; no lactation after confinement; deafness; insomnia; convulsions in children. After a stroke when the patient is inconscious with phlegm coming from the mouth, use the prismatic needle to revive the patient.

Treatment: Needle: 1/16 inch.
Moxa: 1 to 3 times.

Stimulus: Local pain stimulus.

22.2 **Hou Hsi** *back stream* **SI-3**

Location: On the outside edge of the hand, behind the metacarpophalangeal joint of the little finger.

Effects: Malaria with cold sensations and high fevers; jaundice; night sweating; excessive sweating; stiffness of the neck; cramping of the arm and elbow; conjunctivitis with a film over the eye; deafness; epistaxis; madness; epilepsy; scabies.

Treatment: Needle: 1/8 to 1/4 inch.
Moxa: 1 to 3 times.

Stimulus: Down the small finger.

Note: To locate and treat this point, slightly clench the hand; the point is on the cleft where the finger and palm meet.

22.3 **Wan Gu** *wrist bone* **SI-4**

Location: Outside edge of the hand between the proximal end of the metacarpal and the wrist bones.

Effects: High fever without perspiration; headache; swollen neck; jaundice; ringing in the ear; malaria; uncontrollable streams of cold tears with a film on the eyes; convulsions and cramping in children; paralysis of arm and elbow, arm cannot bend or straighten; cramping and/or numbness of the five fingers; pain on the outer wrist.

Treatment: Needle: 1/4 inch.
Moxa: 3 times.

Stimulus: Around the wrist.

Note: To locate this point, use your fingernail to press from SI-3 along the outside edge of the hand until it touches the wrist bone, the point is located on the front of the wrist bone.

Note: To treat this point, have the patient make a fist, then either rest the thumb down on the table, or if the patient has wrist pain, rest the elbow on the table and hold the forearm vertically.

22.4 **Yang Guu** *yang valley* **SI-5**

Location: Outside edge of arm between the ulnar and wrist bone; behind SI-4, 1/2 division.

Effects: Madness; high temperature without perspiration; swollen neck; stiffness; tinnitus; toothache; pain on outside edge of arm; delirium with eyes looking left and right; dizziness in eyes; child with cramping and stiffness who cannot drink milk.

Treatment: Needle: almost 1/4 inch.
Moxa: 3 times.

Stimulus: Felt around the wrist bone.

22.5 **Hsiao Hai** *small sea* **SI-8**

Location: Outside of the elbow, in the hollow between the proximal end of the ulnar bone and the distal end of humerus when the elbow is bent at a 90 degree angle.

Effects: Pain on the neck and lower jaw; pain on the shoulder and elbow; pain on gums; swollen neck; pain on the armpit and elbow; pain on the lower abdomen; epilepsy; cramping of the neck; madness with the patient running around crazily; stiffness of the shoulder; deafness; jaundice with yellow eyes.

Treatment: Needle: almost 1/4 inch.
Moxa: 3 times.

Stimulus: Reaction around the elbow.

22.6 **Jhou Jian** *sharp point of elbow* **XA-2**

Location: Tip of the elbow, when the arm is bent 90 degrees, the point is in a small cleft.

Effects: Scrofula; furuncle; general inflammation; inflammation of cecum; carbuncle in cecum.

Treatment: **No Needle.**
Moxa: 7 to 15 times; after three days or seven days, repeat, until done a total of 100 times.

Stimulus: Up the arm; strongest reaction up to the neck.

Note: To locate this point, bend the arm at an angle of 90 degrees.

22.7 **Jung Kuei** *middle leader* **XFi-2**

Location: The yang side of the middle finger, at the center of the second knuckle. Bend the finger, a small hollow is on top of the knuckle.

Effects: Belching; hiccoughs; severe vomiting.

Treatment: **No Needle.**
Moxa: 5 to 7 times, 1/3 rice grain size.

Stimulus: Up and down the finger a distance of one inch.

22.8 **Dah Shiao Guu Kung** *big and small hollows of the bone* **XFi-3**

Location: 1) Dah guu kung: a little distal to the center of the second knuckle of the thumb. 2) Shiao guu kung: a little distal to the center of the second knuckle of the little finger.

Effects: Cataracts; excessive lacrymation; film on the eyes; itching of the eyes; pain and arthritis on respective knuckles.

Treatment: **No Needle.**
Moxa: 7 times, 1/3 rice grain size.

Stimulus: Down to the tip of finger or thumb.

22.9 **Bah Hsieh** *eight ghosts* **XHn-1**

Location: There are four main points on each hand, the first is LI-4. The others are found 2/5 division distal to the depressions between the ends of the first finger knuckles. You can also needle proximal to the same knuckle depressions, to take the place of needling the first series. In severe conditions, use all seven points, these points include TW-2 and TW-3.

Effects: Headache; toothache; conjunctivitis; inflammation on the arm; all fingers numb and painful; itching on the palm; stiffness and/or pain of the knuckles.

Treatment: Needle: 1/8 to 1/4 inch.
Moxa: 5 times.

Stimulus: Down to the fingers.

Note: To locate this point, have the patient clench the hand.

22.10 **Sih Shuian** *ten drain off* **XFi-4**

Location: On the ten fingers, where the middle of the fingernail meets the finger.

Effects: Stroke; sunstroke; tonsillitis; sudden madness; typhoid fever; severe high temperature.

Treatment: Needle: 1/8 inch. Use a thicker needle; bleed the point until the dark blood is gone and fresh blood comes out.
No Moxa.

Stimulus: Severe local pain stimulus.

22.11 **Wu Fu** *five tigers* **XFi-5**

Location: In the middle of the second knuckles of the four fingers and thumb.

Effects: Stiffness of the five fingers, cannot straighten or bend; pain on the five fingers.

Treatment: **No Needle.**
Moxa: 3 to 5 times, 1/2 rice grain size.

Stimulus: Down to tip of fingers, thumb.

22.12 **Wen Tao** *tip of crease* **XFi-6**

Location: When the hand is clenched, these points are at the end of all the major finger creases, on the edges of the fingers. Therefore, there are four points on each finger, two on each thumb.

Effects: Stiff and painful finger joints.

Treatment: Needle: 1/8 to 1/4 inch.
Moxa: 3 to 5 times, sesame size.

Stimulus: Felt down the middle of the palm side of the fingers.

Section 23 **Spleen Meridian**

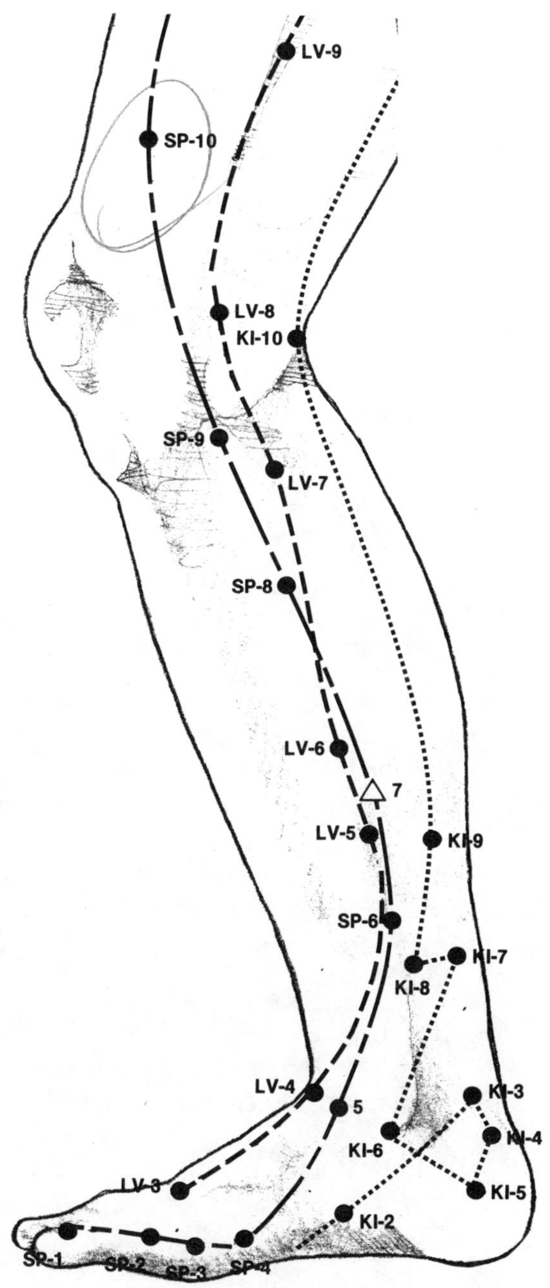

Spleen Meridian

Illustration 25

23.1 **Yin Bai** *hidden white* **SP-1**

Location: The inside corner of the big toe nail.

Effects: Pleurisy (swelling of the abdomen, panting and insomnia); hot sensations in the chest; vomiting and anorexia; diarrhea; epilepsy; patient unconscious; severe hemorrhaging from the uterus; excessive menstruation; hypertension; insomnia; severe vomiting and diarrhea in children.

Treatment: Needle: 1/16 inch.
Moxa: 3 times, 1/3 rice grain size.

Stimulus: Severe, local pain.

23.2 **Dah Du** *big capital* **SP-2**

Location: On the inside edge of the foot, the second depression distal to the metatarsophalangeal joint.

Effects: High fever without perspiration; difficulty lying down; general neurasthenia; body heavy and joints painful; after the flu, encroaching cold feelings moving up the four limbs; full feeling in the chest and abdomen, with vomiting; gastric pain; dizziness on the eyes; lumbago; difficulty bending forwards and backwards; constipation; four limbs swollen; cramping in children; hemorrhage of the uterus; menorrhalgia.

Treatment: Needle: 1/8 inch.
Moxa: 5 times. **No Moxa** during pregnancy or for three months after confinement.

Stimulus: Felt to the end of the big toe.

Note: Locate this point by sliding your fingernail from the joint towards the toe. The second depression is the point. To treat this point, it is not necessary to have the foot flat on the floor.

23.3 **Gung Sun** *grandfather grandson* **SP-4**

Location: On the inside edge of the foot, one division behind the metatarsophalangeal joint, under the metatarsal bone, where the yin and yang skin meet.

Effects: Pericarditis; pleurisy; stomach cancer; vomiting; stomachache; overcooling in the spleen; decreased appetite; pain of the lower abdomen; intestinal hemorrhage; epilepsy; melancholia and crazed speech; retained placenta; head, face swollen; dropsy; gas; enlargement of the abdomen; cholera.

Treatment: Needle: 1/3 inch.
Moxa: 3 times.

Stimulus: Stimulus felt about three inches up and down spleen line.

Note: It is not necessary to place the foot flat on the floor to treat this point.

23.4 **Shang Chiu** *merchant hill* **SP-5**

Location: Anterior to the medial malleolus approximately 1/2 division, in the hollow posterior to the tendon.

Effects: Gas; enlargement of the abdomen; borborygmi; vomiting; constipation; diarrhea; indigestion; severe gastric pain; piles; jaundice; weakness of the spleen and the patient is unhappy; sighing; sadness in heart and mind; excessive thinking; patient's body feels heavy and the joints are painful; patient feels lazy and sleepy; pain of the inner thigh; inner foot pain; bone cancer; tongue stiff and painful; child with severe vomiting and diarrhea; whooping cough.

Treatment: Needle: 1/4 inch.
Moxa: 3 times.

Stimulus: Reaction felt to the big toe.

Note: To treat and locate this point the foot should be placed flat on the floor, the knee bent at a 90 degree angle with the foot not turned either to the left or to the right, and the needle inserted perpendicular to the point.

23.5 **San Yin Jiao** *three yin crossing* **SP-6**

Location: Three divisions up proximal to the upper edge of medial malleolus, 1/4 inch behind the tibia.
Note: The three yin meridians of the leg - kidney, liver and spleen, cross at this point.

Effects: Weakness of the spleen and stomach; gas, enlargement of stomach; poor appetite; borborygmi; sticky and undigested stools; after eating, vomiting of stomach liquid; intestinal pain; dysuria; bedwetting; anuria; pain under the umbilicus; pain in the penis; gonorrhea; wet dreams; spermatorrhea; inflammation of a testicle; sexual intercourse during menstruation preceding gradual emaciation of the female; abdominal tumor; menorrhalgia; increased duration of menstrual period, with a scanty flow; menstrual cramps; baby dies in the womb; difficult labor; after confinement, blood trapped in the uterus; excessive bleeding after confinement; patient anemic after confinement; severe hemorrhaging of the uterus; patient unconscious; baby moves too much in the uterus; white and red vaginal discharge; four limbs tired and cold; lower limbs painful and/or numb; pain of the inner side of the knee; hypertension; insomnia; coughing; edema.

Treatment: Needle: 1/4 to 1/2 inch.
No Needle if patient is pregnant.
Moxa: 3 to 5 times.

Stimulus: Down to the inner ankle and big toe.

Note: To treat this point, place the foot flat on the floor, stool, etc. If the foot is turned left or right, correct stimulus will not be obtained.

23.6 **Yin Ling Chuan** *yin hill stream* **SP-9**

Location: On the inner corner of the proximal edge of the tibia, with the knee bent in a 90 degree angle.

Effects: Cholera; overcooling in the stomach; anorexia; indigestion; diarrhea; dropsy; loins swollen; panting; difficulty lying down; lumbago, and difficulty bending forwards and backwards; acute or chronic knee inflammation; dysuria; bed-wetting; wet dreams; inflammation of the vagina; insomnia.

Treatment: Needle: 1/4 to 1/2 inch.
Moxa: 3 to 5 times.

Stimulus: Felt up to the knee and down the leg about three inches.

23.7 **Sheue Hai** *sea of blood* **SP-10**

Location: With the knee bent at 90 degree angle, the point is two divisions proximal to the upper edge of the patella, on the medial side of the leg. Imagine a rectangular leg; this point would then be at the anterior inside corner.

Effects: Pleurisy; stomach enlarged; chi moving up; dysmenorrhea; menorrhagia; metritis; red and white vaginal discharge; gonorrhea; itching in the scrotum; scrotum swollen with fluid; itching; abscess; all skin diseases.

Treatment: Needle: 1/4 to 1/2 inch.
Moxa: 3 to 5 times.

Stimulus: Down to the knee and up the meridian 2 to 3 inches.

Note: To locate this point have the patient sitting with the knee bent at a 90 degree angle.

Section 24 **Liver Meridian**

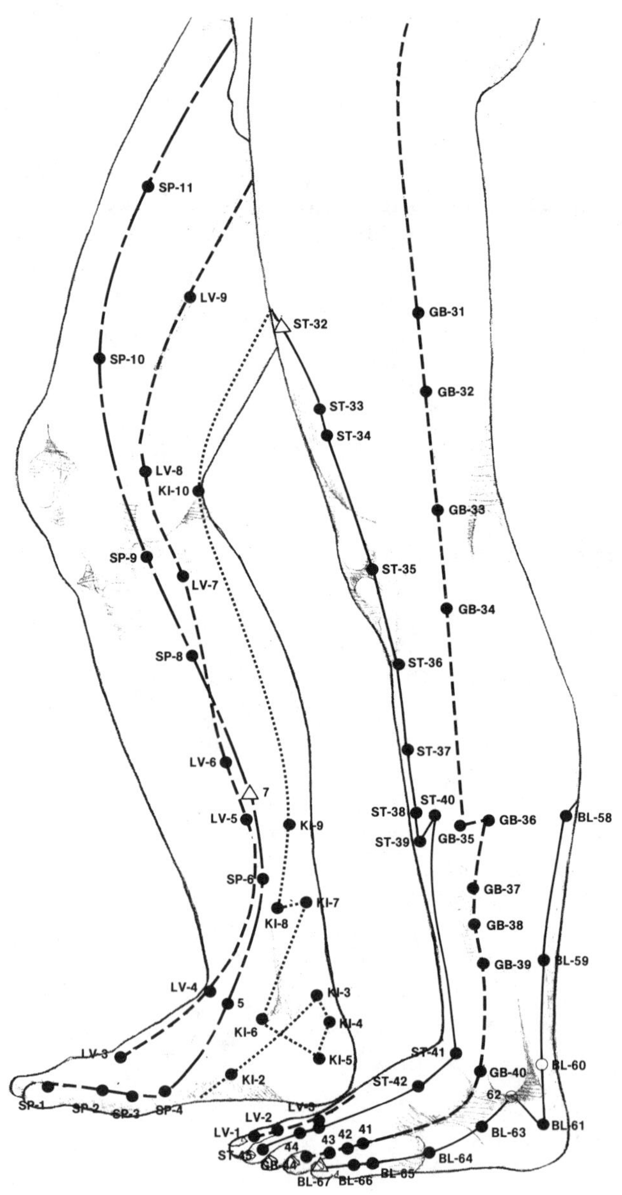

Liver Meridian
Illustration 26

24.1 **Da Duen** *big heap* **LV-1**

Location: Behind the outer corner of the big toe nail.

Effects: Swollen abdomen; lower abdomen painful; intestinal pain; constipation; bed-wetting; frequent urination; diabetes; gonorrhea; hernia; inflammation of the testicles; scrotum swollen; pain in the penis; cramping of the penis; menorrhagia; extensive menstrual period with scanty flow; severe hemorrhaging of the uterus; vaginal pain; convulsions in a child; patient suddenly faints as if dying; patient sleeps too much.

Treatment: Needle: 1/16 inch.
Moxa: 3 times.

Stimulus: Severe local pain.

Note: According to the old books, this point is behind the toe where the hair grows. This is incorrect.

24.2 **Shing Jian** *walk in between* **LV-2**

Location: In between the big and second toe, half-way between the web and the joint.

Effects: Hemoptysis; chest and sides painful; pain at the end of the sternum; lower abdomen swollen; intestinal pain; constipation; hernia; bedwetting; dysuria; diabetes; lumbago; difficulty bending forwards and backwards; knee pain; four limbs with encroaching cold feelings; sighing; convulsions in children; night-blindness; excessive tearing; heavy feeling of the eyelids; menorrhagia; excessive hemorrhaging from the uterus; extensive duration of the menstrual cycle with scanty flow.

Treatment: Needle: 1/4 inch.
Moxa: 3 times.

Stimulus: Reaction felt to the toe.

24.3 **Tai Chung** *bigger rushing* **LV-3**

Location: 1 and 1/2 divisions proximal to the metatarsophalangeal joints, between the first and second metatarsal.

Effects: Hemoptysis; swollen legs; patient frightened and lacks chi; vomiting and body feels cold; dry throat with thirst; lips swollen; upper abdomen and sides swollen; pain in the area below the sternum; angina pectoris; swollen lower abdomen; pain from the lumbar area reaching the lower abdomen; bedwetting; dysuria; constipation; diarrhea; hernia; retraction of testicle; pain in the genitals; amenorrhea; menorrhagia; after confinement, excessive bleeding; soreness of the tibia; pain on the medial malleolus; feet cold; convulsions in children; numb throat.

Treatment: Needle: 1/2 inch.
Moxa: 3 times.
There is a big pulse close to this point.

Stimulus: Up the higher part of the foot, down to the toes.

24.4 **Jung Feng** *middle seal* **LV-4**

Location: Approximately one division anterior to the medial malleolus, in between the two tendons.

Effects: Cattarh of the bladder; gonorrhea; dysuria; difficult defecation; lower abdomen swollen; male genitals retracted into the body; spermatorrhea; body numbness; pain of the five toes; pain on ankle joints; patient has difficulty walking.

Treatment: Needle: 1/4 inch or a little more.
Moxa: 3 times.

Stimulus: Down to the five toes.

24.5 **Shi Guan** *knee gate* **LV-7**

Location: Two divisions distal to SP-9, one division posterior to the inner edge of the tibia, between two muscles; by the old book, this point is just one division down from SP-9.

Effects: Numbness of the knee; knee painful, difficult to straighten or bend; pain on the inner side of the foreleg; pain in the throat.

Treatment: Needle: 1/2 inch or a little more.
Moxa: 5 times.

Stimulus: Felt on the inner side of the calf.

Note: Bend the knee to a 90 degree angle to locate and treat this point.

24.6 **Chu Chuan** *crooked spring* **LV-8**

Location: On the inner side of the knee, with the knee bent so that the foot touches the thigh; the point is found by pressing down from the meeting of the two bones, to the hollow. Note: The point is not necessarily at the end of the knee crease.

Effects: Pain on the knee; cramping of the knee, difficult to bend or stretch; pain of the inner thigh; cold feelings on the shins; difficulty lifting the four limbs; swelling of the abdomen and loins; swelling of the lower abdomen; lower abdominal pain; diarrhea, with a lot of liquid; dysentery with pus and blood; anuria; penis pain; sexual organs swollen; spermatorrhea; itching in the vagina; prolapse of the uterus; bleeding from the anus; epistaxis.

Treatment: Needle: 1/2 to 3/4 inch.
Moxa: 3 times.

Stimulus: Felt on the inside of the knee and up the thigh.

Note: To locate this point, bend the knee so that the foot touches the thigh. Treat with the knee flexed.

Section 25 **Kidney Meridian**

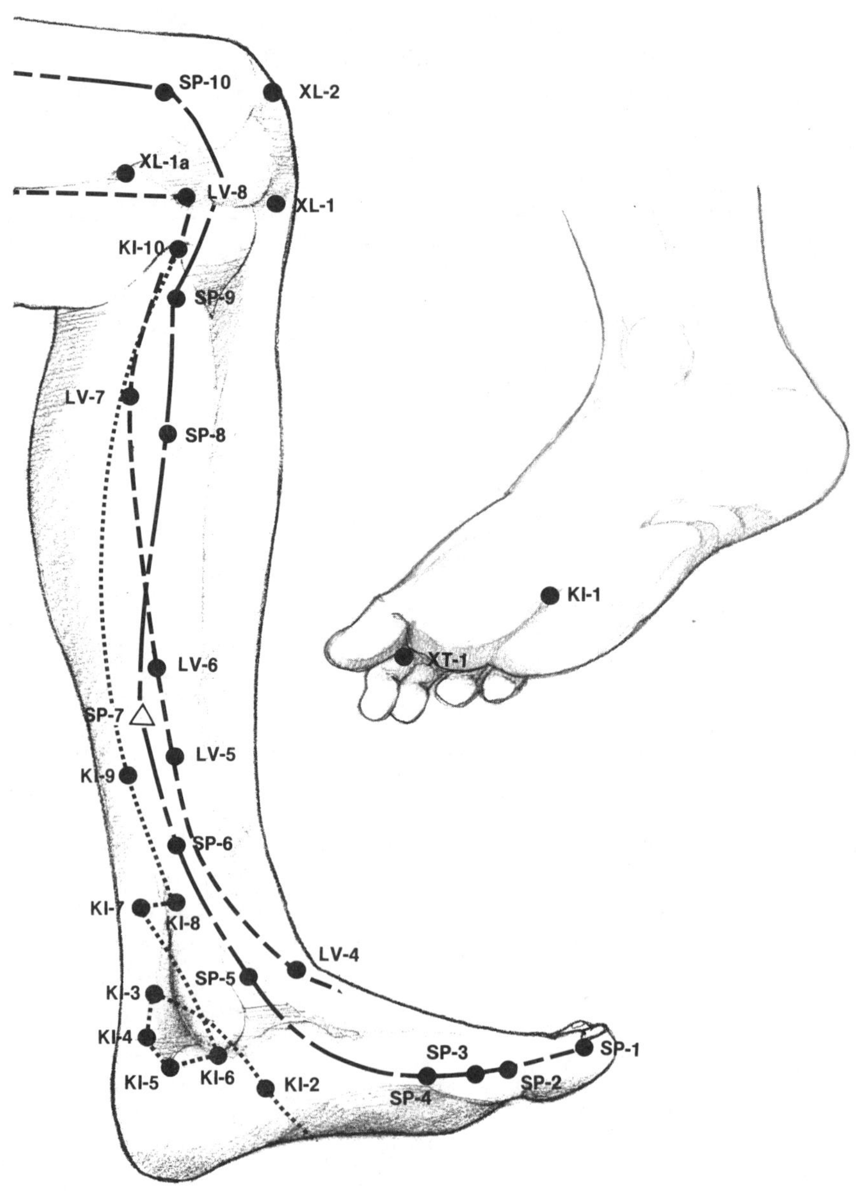

Kidney Meridian
Illustration 27

25.1 **Yung Chuan** *bubbling up spring* **KI-1**

Location: On the distal half of the sole of the foot where the midline of the sole intersects a line level to the bottom edge of the big toe metatarsophalangeal joint. Or, you can find the point by pressing with the fingernail down the midline of the sole of the foot, from the top of the foot. The first depression is the point.

Effects: Patient fainting with a darkened face; tuberculosis; coughing with a little blood; severe headache; head feels like it's going to explode; blood congested; meningitis; epistaxis; angina pectoris; crying; patient frightened, fearful of being captured; hot sensations in the chest; melancholia in chest; heart palpitations; full feeling in the chest and abdomen; epilepsy; tonsillitis; a swollen throat, with dyspnea; tongue stiff; loss of voice; sudden muteness; cramping of the whole body; cramping in cholera; diarrhea with heavy feelings in anus; lumbago; difficulty defecating; swollen abdomen, with lumbago; dysuria; hernia; during pregnancy, sudden anuria; abdomen swollen with worms, or gas, or tumor (female or male); a lump of gas moving inside abdomen; cramp in uterus; woman cannot conceive; numbness of vagina; prolapse of uterus; pain on tibia bone; encroaching coldness from foot to knee; pain of five toes; difficulty stepping on the floor; hot sensations of the sole; pain on inner side of thigh; jaundice; urticaria; excessive sleeping. This point can draw down all overheating from the upper part of the body.

Treatment: Needle: 1/4 inch or a little more.
Moxa: 3 to 5 times.

Stimulus: Reaction down to the five toes with electric sensations.

25.2 **Ran Gu** *blazing valley* **KI-2**

Location: Below the center of the navicular bone.

Effects: Takes away all overheating from the kidneys; inflammation of the larynx and pharynx; tonsillitis; melancholia and full feelings in the chest, with thirst; heart painful (as if it had been stabbed); patient frightened, fearful of being captured; swollen lower abdomen, reaction up to the chest; hemoptysis; bedwetting; continued dribbling after urination; gonorrhea; diabetes; inflammation of the testicles; wet-dreams; excessive perspiration; night-sweating; difficult to conceive; prolapse of the uterus; congestion of the vagina; vaginal itching; swollen ankle joints; painful ankle joints; difficulty to stepping on the floor; shin sore; difficult to stand up; tetanus in children.

Treatment: Needle: 1/4 inch or a little more.
Moxa: 3 times.

Stimulus: Felt forward to the toe.

Note: To treat and locate this point, rest the side of the foot on a chair. Apply some amount of pressure to the pressing finger when needling.

25.3 **Tai Hsi** *bigger stream* **KI-3**

Location: Behind the medial malleolus 1/2 finger division; midway between the edge of the medial malleolus and tendon.

Effects: High fever without perspiration; with "flu" where there is coldness in the four limbs (if the pulse is sinking, there is coldness in the four limbs encroaching on the elbows and knees, the patient will develop panting and die); a patient with little interest in anything except sleeping; vomiting; hiccoughs; very thick gum like phlegm in the mouth; coughing without appetite, either overcooling or overheating; swelling in the throat; spitting with blood; severe angina pectoris; pain in the abdomen and loins; lumbago; constipation; pain in the uterus; sore and painful foot; pain on the heel; pain on the sole of foot.

Treatment: Needle: 1/4 to 1/2 inch.
Moxa: 3 times.

Stimulus: Through the heel to the sole, with electric sensation.

Note: There is a pulse close to this point.

Note: In an adult with a severe disease, if a pulse still beating here, the patient will live, if there is no pulse, the patient will die.

Note: To locate this point, it is not necessary to put the foot on the floor.

25.4 **Jiu Hai** *shining sea* **KI-6**

Location: 1/3 division below medial malleolus, anterior to the big tendon, or between two tendons.

Effects: Tonsillitis; dryness of the throat; four limbs lazy and tired; excessive sleeping; vomiting; pain of the lower abdomen; constipation; irregular menstruation; prolapse of uterus; excessive vaginal secretion during intercourse; itching in the vagina; spasm in the vagina; retained placenta; acute hernia; chronic malaria; stars in vision; foot swollen; ankle joint painful. If epilepsy occurs at night, use moxa on this point.

Treatment: Needle: 1/4 inch or a little more.
Moxa: 3 to 7 times.

Stimulus: Inside ankle joint, or a little forward.

Note: Rest the opposite side of the foot on a chair to locate and treat this point.

25.5 **Da Jung** *big bell* **KI-4**

Location: One half division down from KI-3 and 1/4 division posterior, in front of the tendon.

Effects: Foolishness; palpitations; hot sensations in the mouth; dry tongue; stenosis of the esophagus; sound in the throat during breathing; coughing; vomiting; constipation; gonorrhea; pain on the back and spine; patient likes to sleep excessively; patient frightened and unhappy; cramping in the uterus.

Treatment: Needle: 1/8 to 1/4 inch.
Moxa: 3 times.

Stimulus: Down one side of the heel.

25.6 **Fu Liu** *returning current* **KI-7**

Location: Up 2 divisions from the edge of the inside ankle bone, in front of the edge of the back tendon.

Effects: Gonorrhea; dysuria; constipation; dysentery, white or red; pain in lower abdomen; dropsy; irregular menstruation; amenorrhea; long periods of menstruation; prolapse of the uterus; excessive secretion during sexual intercourse; pain in the inner thigh; pain in the bottom of the heel; night sweats.

Treatment: Needle: 1/4 to 1/2 inch.
Moxa: 3 to 5 times.

Stimulus: The reaction is felt to the bottom of the heel with electric sensation.

Note: To locate this point put the foot squarely on the table; the needle should be inserted at a 45 degree angle toward the tibia bone.

25.7 **Jao Shin** *exchanging letters* **KI-8**

Location: Proximal from the edge of the medial malleolus 2 divisions, behind the tibia 1/2 division, between two small muscles.

Effects: Inflammation of the spine; back pain; difficulty bending forwards and backwards; the patient loses control over the foot and is unable to raise it up; beri-beri; pain under the heel; pleurisy; dropsy (KI-7); borborygmi; pain in abdomen; swelling of abdomen; night sweats; excessive sweating; after the "flu" with no sweating; malaria; piles; dryness of the mouth; overheating in the stomach; worms moving in the stomach and excessive saliva in the mouth; quick anger and excessive talking; sudden cessation of the pulse (use with LI-4 and PC-5.)

Treatment: Needle: 1/2 to 3/4 inch.
Moxa: 5 to 7 times.

Stimulus: Reaction through the heel to the big toe, with electric sensations.

Note: To locate this point, the foot should be placed squarely on the floor. The needle should be inserted at a 45 degree angle toward the tendon.

Section 26 **Stomach Meridian**

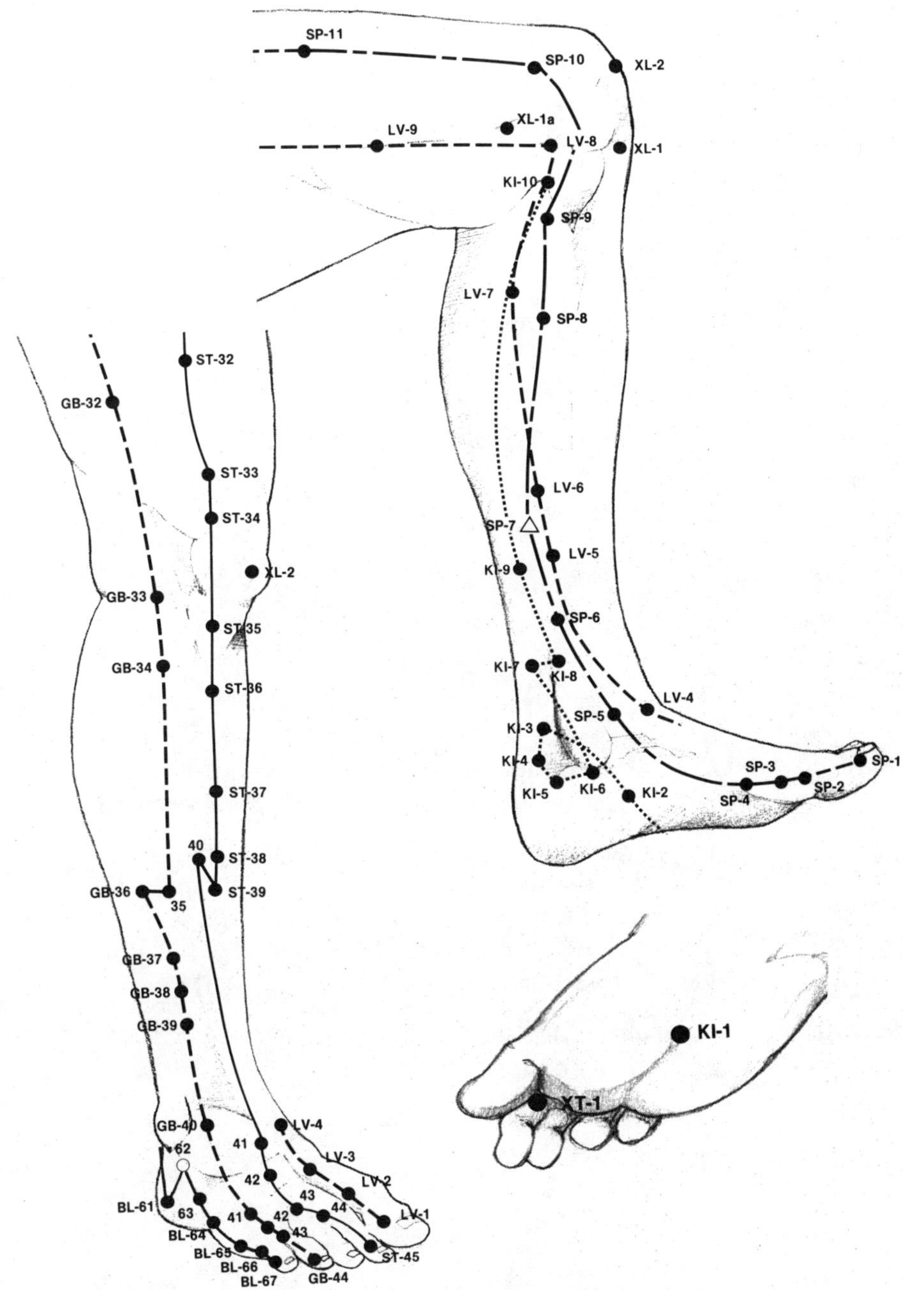

Stomach Meridian

Illustration 28

26.1 **Yin Shih** *yin market* **ST-33**

Location: Three divisions proximal to the top edge of the patella, on the outer corner of the thigh (refer to SP-10).

Effects: Lumbar, thigh, knees are cold like water, numb, cannot straighten and bend; beri-beri; Parkinson's disease (use moxa here and on HT-3;) weakness of the leg; pain and swelling in the abdomen; diabetes; pain in uterus.

Treatment: Needle: 1/4 to 1/2 inch.
Moxa: 3 times.

Stimulus: Reaction down to the knee.

26.2 **Shi Yan** *eyes of the knee* **XL-1**

Location: Under the patella, in two large hollows of both sides of the knee, when knee is bent at a 90 degree angle.

Effects: Inflammation of knee; swelling of knee ("crane knee") ; pain of the knee joint.

Treatment: Needle: 1 and 1/2 to 2 and 1/2 inches.
Moxa: 5 to 7 times.

Stimulus: Felt around the knee joint. The outer eye of the knee reacts up and down the leg.

Note: The outer eye of the knee is ST-35.

26.3 **Shi Yik** *wings of the knee* **XL-1a**

Location: With leg bent at a 90 degree angle: three divisions behind the knee bone proximal from the knee bone to both sides of knee, in the middle of the thigh.

Effects: Pain in the knee.

Treatment: Needle: 1/2 to 3/4 inch.
Moxa: Rarely used at this point.

Stimulus: Reaction down to the knee.

26.4 **Hok Deng** *top of the crane* **XL-2**

Location: In the vertical cleft at the center of the patella. In the center of the cleft.

Effects: Weakness of the knee and leg.

Treatment: **No Needle.**
Moxa: 7 times, half rice grain size.

Stimulus: Reaction down to the foot.

Note: Some acupuncturists treat this point at the upper edge of the patella; this is incorrect.

Note: To locate and treat this point, the leg must be bent at a 90 degree angle.

26.5 **Tsu San Li** *leg three miles* **ST-36**

Location: Distal to the lateral side of the knee. Two divisions distal to the meeting of the tibia and fibula (GB-34); 1/4 division lateral to tibia.

Effects: For every type of stomach and intestinal disease; overheating in the stomach; overcooling in the stomach; swelling of the upper abdomen; poor appetite; cramping in stomach; poor digestion; vomiting; melancholia; acute angina pectoris; gas from stomach rising up; borborygmi; constipation; diarrhea; lower abdomen hard; abdomen swollen with gas; dropsy; hot sensations in the chest; anuria; gonorrhea; hernia; patient cannot stand erect with panting; headache; dizziness; after confinement, excessive bleeding and dizziness; crazy speech; crazy singing; crazy laughing; patient frightened; patient angry and scolding; dimness of the eyes; no perspiration following the flu; overheating with a bitter taste in the mouth; difficulty speaking; numbness of the throat; breast swollen; carbuncle in breast; emaciation due to T.B.; neurasthenia; spitting with blood; lumbago; pain on knee; shin pain; high blood pressure. This point can cure many types of disease. Moxa applied frequently to this point will insure long life.

Treatment: Needle: 1/4 to 1/2 inch.
Moxa: 3 to 7 times, also 100 to 500 times.

Stimulus: Up to the knee, down to end of tibia.

26.6 **Lan Wei** *appendix* **ST-36a**

Location: One division distal to ST-36.

Effects: The same as ST-36; but the effect on these conditions is accentuated at this point; especially powerful for inflammation of the appendix.

Treatment: Same as ST-36.

Stimulus: Same as ST-36.

26.7 **Feng Lung** *abundant bulge* **ST-40**

Location: From the crease behind the knee to the ankle is 16 divisions. The point is 8 divisions proximal to the center of the lateral malleolus, and 1/2 division lateral to the lateral side of the tibia.

Effects: Excessive phlegm; panting; pleurisy; numbness of the throat; sudden muteness; stabbing pain in the chest; cutting pain in the abdomen; difficulty in passing urine and feces; headache; madness; seeing ghosts; excessive laughing; laziness; pain and soreness in thigh and knee; withering of muscles in shin area; drop foot; swelling of four limbs.

Treatment: Needle: 1 and 1/2 to 3 inches (according to size of leg).
Moxa: 3 to 7 times.

Stimulus: Down to the toes and foot; strongest reaction up to the chest.

26.8 **Shye Shi** *loosening stream* **ST-41**

Location: In front of the foot there are three tendons. Between the medial malleolus and the first tendon is SP-5. Lateral to this tendon is LV-4. Lateral to the next tendon is ST-41. Lateral to the last tendon and anterior to the lateral malleolus is GB-40.

Effects: Headache; madness; dizziness in the eyes; red eyes; pain in elbow; redness of the face; swelling of face; darkness of the face; melancholia; crying; cholera; abdomen swollen; a heavy feeling in the anus after bowel movement; cold chi rushing up to chest; thigh cramps; knee and shin cramps.

Treatment: Needle: 1/4 to 1/2 inch.
Moxa: 3 times.

Stimulus: Down to the toes.

26.9 **Chung Yang** *rushing yang* **ST-42**

Location: 1 and 1/2 divisions distal to ST-41. Between second and third metatarsal bones. There is a pulse at this point.

Effects: One side of face paralyzed; pain from tooth decay; chronic madness; abdomen swollen; patient anorexic; front of body painful and weak.

Treatment: Needle: 1/4 inch.
Moxa: 3 times.

Stimulus: Down to the toes.

Note: When treating this point, be careful of the pulse.

26.10 **Nei Ting** *inner courtyard* **ST-44**

Location: Between the second and third toes; halfway between the metatarsophalangeal joint and the web of the toes.

Effects: Toothache; stomachache; menorrhalgia; swelling of the abdomen; cholera; diarrhea; dropsy; paralysis of one side of face; epistaxis; tonsillitis; hatred of human voices; a cold feeling ascending the four limbs; soreness/numbness of the foot; pain on scalp; malaria without appetite.

Treatment: Needle: 1/4 inch.
Moxa: 3 times.

Stimulus: Down to the toe.

Note: To locate this point, bend the toes, find the point between the edge of the web and the joint.

26.11 **Li Dui** *sharpening exchange* **ST-45**

Location: At the outer, lower corner of the second toenail.

Effects: Fainting, patient cannot talk (death-like); excessive fright; excessive sleeping; madness; epistaxis; numbness of the throat; one side of the face paralyzed; toothache; chapped lips; neck and chest swollen, with full feelings in the chest and abdomen; dropsy; swelling of the face; high fever without perspiration; anorexic malaria; pain in the groin; knee pain; cold sensations in the shins; pain from shin to the foot; excessive hunger; yellow urine; hepatitis.

Treatment: Needle: 1/16 inch.
Moxa: 1 time.

Stimulus: Local pain stimulus.

26.12 **Tu Yin** *single yin* **XT-1**

Location: Under the second toe, in the middle of the second crease.

Effects: Angina pectoris; pain in the heart; patient cannot stand; hernia; cramping in the uterus; fetus dies in the uterus; retention of placenta; ovaritis; menorrhalgia; severe hiccoughs; morning sickness (use moxa on this point and on PC-5.)

Treatment: **No Needle.**
Moxa: 7 times, 1/2 rice grain size.

Stimulus: Severe local pain and reaction up to chest.

Note: To locate and treat this point, have the patient rest their heel on a chair. Also, on the second toe, there are a number of creases, and they will differ from patient to patient. You must find the most painful crease.

Section 27 **Bladder Meridian**

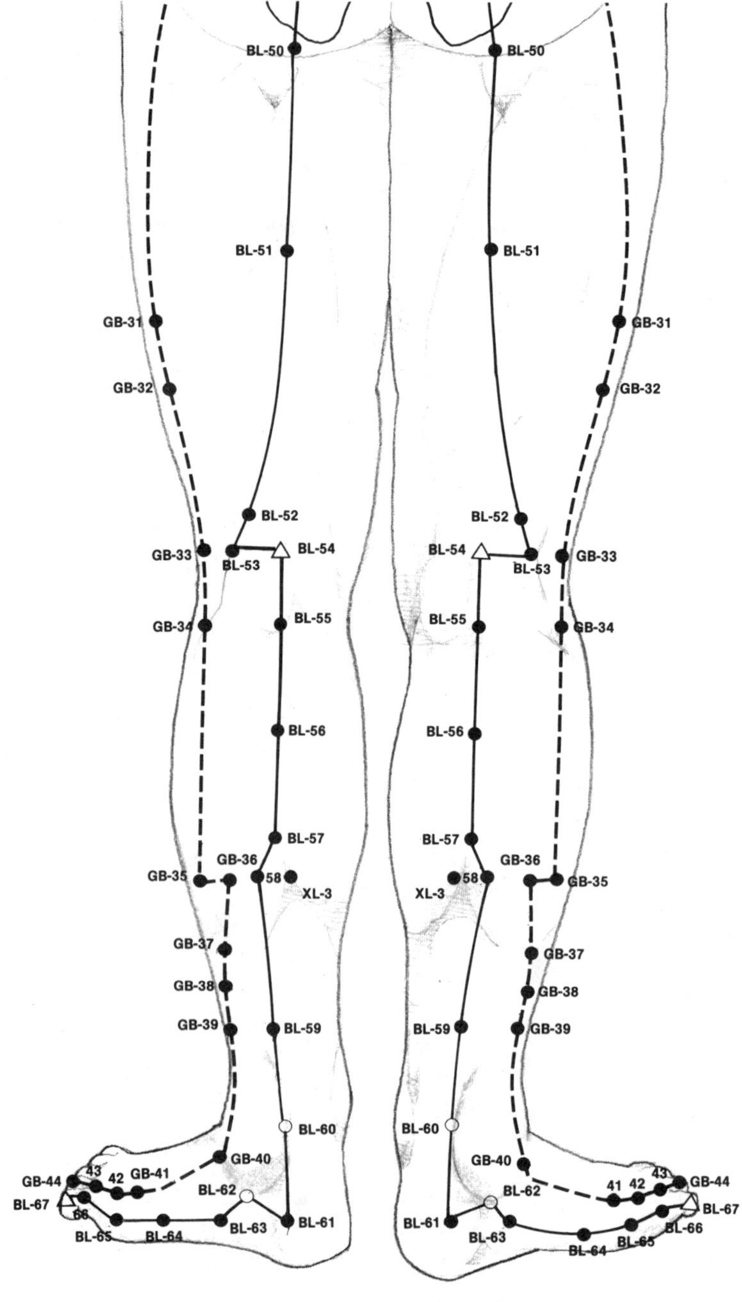

Bladder Meridian

Illustration 29

27.1 **Cheng Fu** *receive and accept* **BL-50**

Location: Where the midline of the back and the thigh intersects the crease beween the buttock and the thigh, between two tendons.

Effects: Pain on the back; swollen buttocks; piles; difficult defecation; dysuria.

Treatment: Needle: 3/4 to 1 inch.
Moxa: 3 to 5 times.

Stimulus: Electric stimulus down to the foot.

27.2 **Wei Jung** *entrusting middle* **BL-54**

Location: In the middle crease behind the knee, between two tendons.

Effects: Four limbs hot after the flu; high fever without perspiration; a cold sensation from the back preceding high fever with profuse sweating; heavy feelings in the head with leg cramps; pain on the back and spine; heavy feelings in the lumbar area; paralysis following stroke; hip joint pain; knee pain, difficult to bend and straighten; legs weak; epistaxis; numbness of the throat; any throat problems; weakness of the body with perspiration; night sweating; anuria; bed-wetting; during heavy winds the hair falls out of eyebrows and head (bleed veins close to this point); any skin disease, abscess or carbuncle; this point takes away body fevers.

Treatment: Needle: 1/2 to 2 inch.
No Moxa.

Stimulus: When needled from 1/2 to 1 inch, a strong electric stimulus to the foot is felt, with the strongest reactions felt in the lumbar area. When needled to 2 inches the reaction is felt behind the patella.

Notes on treating BL-54

Note 1: Moxa here will shorten the nerve, bending the leg permanently, making it difficult for the patient to walk.

Note 2: The best way to locate and treat this point is by having the patient stand up. If the patient cannot stand up, have him lie on his side with his legs straight. If it's difficult to find the two tendons, bend the leg, touch the tendons thereby locating the point. Then restraighten the leg to treat. If the patient has inflammation of the knee and cannot straighten the leg, you can treat the point while the knee is bent, but you must find the two tendons.

Note 3: To treat this point to a depth of two inches, do not insert the needle through the tendons, but to either side of the two tendons. This depth is used only for pain behind the patella. Two inch insertion through the two tendons would be excessive stimulation.

Note 4: Many acupuncture books place this point at the center of the crease behind the knee; this is not correct. Sometimes the two tendons grow a little to the left or a little to the right of center. If you cannot insert the needle through the two tendons, you won't obtain the correct stimulation.

Note 5: Sometimes the patient's nerve is not exactly behind the two tendons. If the needle penetrates up to one inch but there is no stimulation, withdraw the needle and redirect it a little more towards the lateral side of the leg to find the stimulus. If this doesn't work, redirect it towards the inner side of the leg.

27.3 **Cheng Shan** *supporting mountain* **BL-57**

Location: There are 16 divisions between BL-54 and the lateral malleolus; this point is eight divisions below BL-54, in the center of the back of the calf between two muscles.

Effects: For the cramping of the entire body, or only part of the body; lumbago; shaking of the body; beri-beri; sore shins; heel pain; cholera cramping; lockjaw in children; syphilitic buboes; piles; anal hemmorrhaging; gonorrhea; constipation; madness; malaria.

Treatment: Needle: 1/2 to 3/4 inch.
Moxa: 5 times.

Stimulus: Down to the foot, usually with electric sensations.

Note: To locate and treat this point, let the patient stand on the other leg; bend the leg, with the toes touching the floor, tell the patient to relax the leg. Needle at 75 degree angle from the horizontal.

27.4 **Shan Sha** *below the mountain* **XL-3**

Location: Distal to BL-57 one division.

Effects: Chronic inflammation of the testicles; hernia.

Treatment: **No Needle.**
Moxa: 10 times, red bean size.

Stimulus: Reaction down to the heel.

27.5 **Kuen Lun** *Kuen Lun mountain* **BL-60**

Location: Posterior to the lateral malleolus 1/2 division; between the edge of the ankle and the tendon.

Effects: Severe headache on top of the head: dizziness; eye dizziness with severe pain; pain from the chest reacting to the back; coughing; stiffness of the shoulder and back; pain on the spine/back; sciatica; beri-beri; foot swollen; cannot walk; hardness behind the knees; severe ankle pain; epilepsy in children; retained placenta; difficult labor.

Treatment: Needle: 1/4 inch. **No Needle** for pregnant woman. Moxa: 3 times.

Stimulus: Down to the foot and small toes.

Note: Place the foot squarely on the chair to locate and treat this point.

27.6 **Shen Mo** *extended meridian* **BL-62**

Location: 1/2 division below the center of the lateral malleolus, between two small tendons.

Effects: Headache; dizziness; lumbago; lower leg pain; shins sore; difficult to stand up; patient sits down/cannot get up; uterus pain; arteriosclerosis; madness; epilepsy during the daytime (apply three direct moxa).

Treatment: Needle: 1/4 inch.
No Moxa.

Stimulus: Straight down and into the ankle joint.

27.7 **Jin Men** *golden gate* **BL-63**

Location: One division below BL-62, and 1/2 division distal. Just under the apex of the triangular bone.

Effects: Cramping from colera; cramping in part of the body; cramping in children; acute hernia; shock; epilepsy; forehead pain; lower abdomen cramping; peritonitis; shins sore; shaking; cannot stand for a long time; beri-beri; deafness; malaria.

Treatment: Needle: 1/4 inch.
Moxa: 3 times.

Stimulus: Towards the toes, two to three inches from this point.

27.8 **Jih Yin** *extremity of yin* **BL-67**

Location: On the lower outside corner of the small toenail.

Effects: For a breach birth use seven moxa on this point to correct the baby's position. Headaches; stuffed nose; film on eyes; eyes painful; inner canthus painful; melancholia; moving pains over chest and sides; cramps; overcooling malaria (no sweating); dysuria; spermatorrhea; hot sensations under the sole.

Treatment: Needle: 1/16 inch.
Moxa: 1 to 7 times, **No Moxa** for pregant women.

Stimulus: Local pain stimulus.

Section 28 **Gall Bladder Meridian**

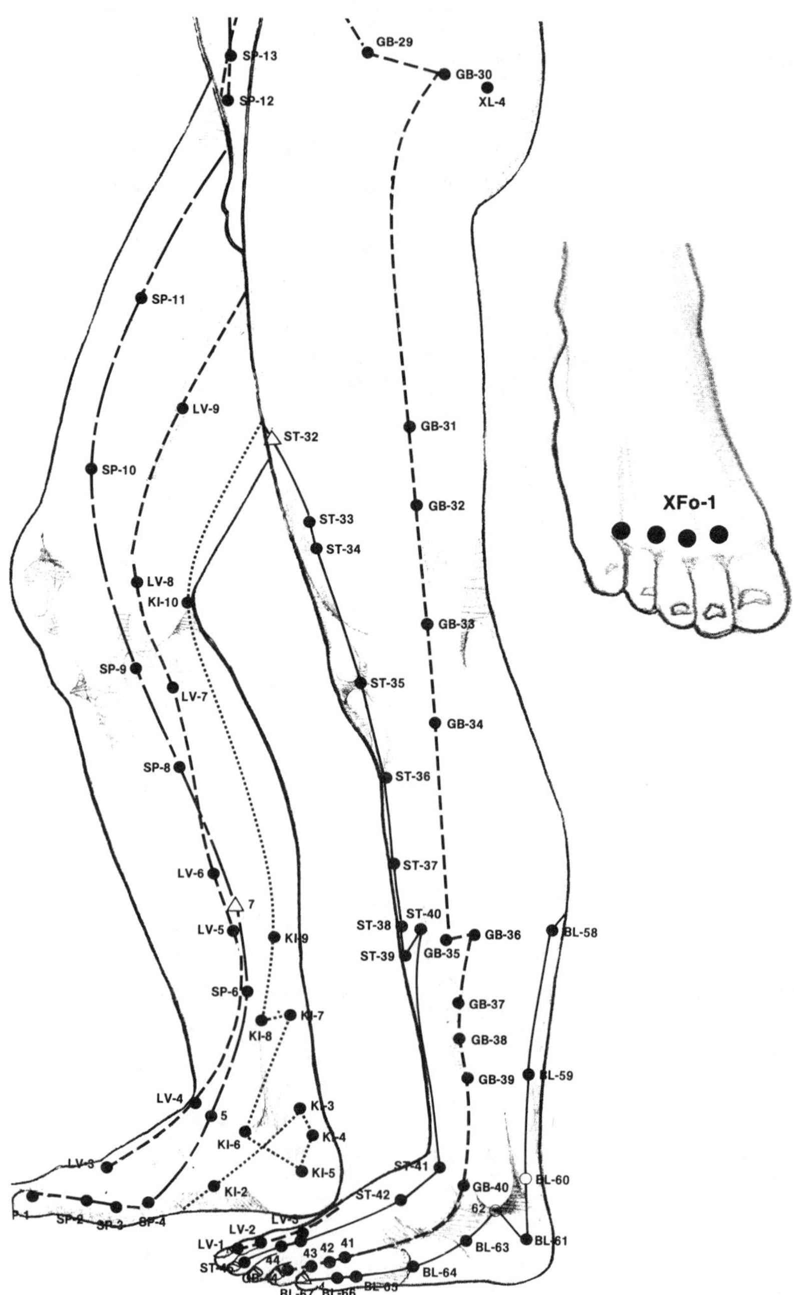

Gall Bladder Meridian

Illustration 30

28.1 **Huan Tiao** *jumping circle* **GB-30**

Location: The patient should lie on one side, with the top leg bent so that the thigh is close to the abdomen. The point is at the edge of the round shaped bone which faces the tip of the butt.

Effects: Sciatica; lumbago reacting to the knee; patient has difficulty turning the body and straightening the leg; hemiplegia; urticaria of the entire body; inflammation of the hip joint.

Treatment: Needle: 1 to 1 and 1/2 inches.
Moxa: 3 to 10 times.

Stimulus: Halfway down the thigh.

Note: To locate and treat this point, have the patient lie on the side with the leg bent to the abdomen. While treating, the needle should just touch the edge of the bone.

28.2 **Huan Jung** *middle of the circle* **XL-4**

Location: 1 and 1/2 divisions toward the tip of the buttock from GB-30.

Effects: Sciatica; whole leg painful.

Treatment: Needle: 1 to 1 and 1/2 inches.
Moxa: 5 times.

Stimulus: Electric stimulus down to the foot.

28.3 **Feng Shi** *wind market* **GB-31**

Location: When the patient is standing up and the arms are hanging straight down, the point is where the end of the middle finger touches the side of the thigh, 7 divisions up from the knee crease.

Effects: Severe beri-beri affecting the heart; weakness of the thigh and knee; lumbago; paralysis; arthritis of the leg and knee; numbness of the leg; itching or numbness of the whole body.

Treatment: Needle: 1/2 inch or a little more.
Moxa: 5 times.

Stimulus: Reaction down to the knee.

28.4 **Yang Guan** *knee yang gate* **GB-33**

Location: From the outer eye of the knee, lateral two divisions, between the femur and tibia. To locate and treat this point, bend the leg so that the calf touches the thigh; the point is at the hollow between and behind the two bones.

Effects: Numbness of the leg; inability to bend or straighten the knee joint; inflammation and/or swelling of the knee.

Treatment: Needle: 1 to 1 and 1/2 inches.
No Moxa.

Stimulus: Stimulus up the thigh, down the calf.

28.5 **Yang Ling Chuan** *yang hill spring* **GB-34**

Location: At the cleft between the proximal ends of the tibia and fibula.

Effects: Hemiplegia; lumbago; sciatica; cramping of the leg; cramping from cholera; inability to bend or straighten the knee; inflammation of the knee ("Crane knee"); thigh numb; coldness, numbness of the whole leg and foot; intercostal neuralgia; constipation; head and face swollen.

Treatment: Needle: 1/4 to 1/2 inch.
Moxa: 7 times.

Stimulus: Reaction is up to the knee and down to the foot.

Note: Bend the leg in a 90 degree angle to treat this point.

28.6 **Yang Fu** *yang support* **GB-38**

Location: Four divisions proximal to the upper edge of the lateral malleolus, between the tibia and fibula.

Effects: Lumbago; lumbar area cold and sore as if sitting in cold water; knee inflammation; leg stiffness; shins sore; legs numb; pain from thigh to ankle; pain on chest and sides; pain moving over body joints; area under armpits swollen; throat numb; excessive perspiration; body shaking.

Treatment: Needle: 3/4 to 1 and 1/4 inches.
Moxa: 3 times.

Stimulus: Reaction down to the toes.

28.7 **Shuan Jung or Jueh Gu** *suspended bell* **GB-39**

Location: Three divisions proximal to lateral malleolus; 1/4 division lateral from vertical line drawn through GB-38.

Effects: Swollen chest and abdomen; hot sensations in the stomach; patient anorexic; sorrowful thoughts; chest painful when coughing; throat numb; neck stiff; epistaxis; nostrils dry; beri-beri; hemiplegia following stroke; lumbago; shin pain; leg and foot cramping; drop foot; dysuria and difficulty defecating; piles.

Treatment: Needle: 3/4 to 1 and 1/4 inches (perpendicular to shin)
Moxa: 5 times.

Stimulus: Down to lateral malleolus, small toes and big toes.

28.8 **Chiu Shu** *hill market* **GB-40**

Location: 1/2 division anterior to the anterior edge of the lateral malleolus, in the hollow posterior to the tendon.

Effects: Chest and sides full and painful, with dyspnea; area under the armpits swollen; dyspnea; lumbar and thigh painful; hip joint painful; cannot stand up after sitting down; neck swollen; film over iris; acute hernia; calf cramping.

Treatment: Needle: 1/4 to 1/2 inch.
Moxa: 5 times.

Stimulus: Felt down to the small toes.

28.9 **Chiao Yin** *foot hole of the yin* **GB-44**

Location: At the outer corner of the fourth toenail.

Effects: Chest and sides painful; coughing with dyspnea; headache with melancholia; throat numb; tongue stiff; mouth dry; hands and feet hot without perspiration; legs cramping; carbuncles on the body; elbow difficult to bend; acute eye dimness; eyes painful; outer canthus painful.

Treatment: Needle: 1/16 inch.
Moxa: 3 times.

Stimulus: Local severe pain.

28.10 **Ba Feng** *eight winds* **XFo-1**

Location: In between the five toes; halfway between the metatarsophalangeal joints and the end of the web of the toes (includes LV-2, ST-44, and GB-43).

Effects: Beri-beri; foot swollen; foot inflamed; foot and toes stiff.

Treatment: Needle: 1/4 inch.
Moxa: 5 times.

Stimulus: Down to the toes.

28.11 **Wah Toh Jet Jih**

Wah Toh's Extra Spleen Point **XSP-1**

Location: On both sides of the spine between two vertebrae at the edges of the body of the cervical, thoracic and lumbar vertebrae about one half division from the center line.

Effects: For spine stiffness, pain or numbness; curved spine (scoliosis).

Treatment: Needle: 1/4 to 1/2 inch for the cervical and thoracic vertebrae and 1/2 to 3/4 inch for the lumbar vertebrae.
Moxa: Direct or indirect.

Stimulus: Lateral across the back from the point used.

Note: Never use all these points at once. Use points at the site of the problem.

Note: For curved spine (scoliosis); if the vertebrae curve to the left treat these points on the left; if the vertebrae curve to the right treat these points to the right.

Points By Meridian

Meeting, Control and Alarm Points

Eight Meeting Points

- The chi meets at CV-17
- The solid organs meet at LV-13
- The hollow organs meet at CV-12
- The blood meets at BL-17
- The pulse meets at LU-9
- The nerves meet at GB-34
- The blood marrow meets at GB-39
- The bones meet at BL-11

Five Controlling Points

The following points control these areas of the body. For problems in these areas you may treat the corresponding points.

- ST-36 for the whole abdominal area
- LU-7 for the head and neck area
- BL-54 for the back area
- PC-6 for the chest to navel area
- LI-4 for the face and mouth

Twelve Mo (Alarm) Points

- Heart CV-14
- Liver LV-14
- Spleen LV-13
- Small Intestine CV-4
- Gallbladder GB-24
  (Note: One rib below LV-14 on the nipple line)
- Stomach CV-12
- Lung LU-1
- Kidney GB-25
  (Note: Under the tip of the twelfth rib on the back)
- Pericardium PC-1
  (Note: One division lateral to the nipple, between the ribs.)
- Large Intestine ST-25
- Bladder CV-3
- Triple Warmer CV-5

If disease strikes one organ in particular you can use these related points if others do not work.

Section 29 **Conception Vessel Meridian**

29.1 **Yu Tang** *jade hall* **CV-18**

Location: On the median line, one intercostal space above CV-17; traditionally 1 and 3/8 divisions above CV-17, between the 3rd and 4th rib bones.

Effects: Chest painful; coughing; chi rushing up; pleurisy; vomiting cold phlegm; full chest; dyspnea; hemoptysis.

Treatment: Needle: 1/4 inch.
Moxa: 5 times.

Stimulus: Felt deep inside the chest.

29.2 **Zi Gung** *purple palace* **CV-19**

Location: On the median line, one intercostal space (1 and 3/8 divisions) above CV-18; that is, at the second intercostal space.

Effects: Painful chest; coughing; dyspnea; bronchitis; vomiting of thick phlegm; breasts swollen and painful; melancholia in the chest; food and drink do not descend; vomiting food; vomiting blood.

Treatment: Needle: 1/4 inch.
Moxa: 7 times.

Stimulus: Felt deep inside the chest.

29.3 **Hua Gai** *splendid covering* **CV-20**

Location: One intercostal space above CV-19 (1 and 3/8 divisions); at the first intercostal space.

Effects: Chest swollen and painful; coughing; swollen numb throat; tonsillitis; unable to swallow food and liquids; asthma. (According to Felix Mann; this point is also effective in stopping smoking).

Treatment: Needle: 1/4 inch.
Moxa: 5 times.

Stimulus: Deep inside the chest and a little up and down from the point.

29.4 **Xuan Ji** *pearl and jade* **CV-21**

Location: One intercostal space above CV-20 (1 and 3/8 divisions), between the clavicle and first rib bones.

Effects: Sides of the chest full and painful; coughing; dyspnea; throat numb/swollen; tonsillitis; inability to swallow liquids.

Treatment: Needle: 1/4 inch.
Moxa: 5 times.

Stimulus: To both sides of the point.

Note: To locate all of the above four points; the patient should be lying down, face up.

Section 30 **Governing Vessel Meridian**

30.1 **Shuan Shu** *suspended pivot* **GV-5**

Location: Between the first and second lumbar vertebra (13th vertebra).

Effects: Loins and back stiff/painful; indigestion; loose stools; frequent urination.

Treatment: Needle: 1/2 inch.
Moxa: 3 to 5 times.

Stimulus: Felt down the spine 2 to 3 vertebrae.

30.2 **Ji Jung** *middle of spine* **GV-6**

Location: Between the 11th and 12th thoracic vertebrae.

Effects: Insanity; epilepsy; abdomen distended; anorexia; jaundice; stomach cramps; hemorrhoids; blood in stools; rectal prolapse in a child.

Treatment: Needle: 1/2 inch.
No Moxa.
Moxa here will cause forward curvature of the spine.

Stimulus: Felt up and down the spine from the point.

30.3 **Jung Shu** *middle pivot* **GV-7**

Location: Between the 10th and 11th thoracic vertebrae.

Effects: Pain in the lower back; stomachache; deterioration of the eyesight.

Treatment: Needle: 1/2 inch.
Moxa: 3 to 5 times.

Stimulus: Up and down the spine.

30.4 **Gin Shu** *contracted nerve* **GV-8**

Location: Between the 9th and 10th vertebrae.

Effects: Insanity; epilepsy; running around madly; rolling of eyes; eyes fixed upwards; cardiac pain; stiffness of the lower back; excessive talking with cardiac pain.

Treatment: Needle: 1/2 inch.
Moxa: 3 to 5 times.

Stimulus: Up and down.

30.5 **Nau Hoo** *brain door* **GV-17**

Location: 4 and 1/2 divisions down from GV-20 on the median line of head.

Effects: **This point is forbidden for needle and moxa.**

Note: Any stimulus of this point will damage the patient's brain causing death.

30.6 **Chiang Jian** *strength in between* **GV-18**

Location: Three divisions below GV-20.

Effects: Severe headaches; vertigo; melancholia; vomiting mucus; epilepsy; depression; neck stiffness; insanity.

Treatment: Needle: 1/8 inch.
Moxa: 5 to 7 times.

Stimulus: Down the back of the head.

30.7 **Dui Duan** *extreme exchange* **GV-27**

Location: At the tip of the philtrum.

Effects: Insanity; delirium; epilepsy; excessive epistaxis; stiff lips; gingivitis; excessive thirst; dry tongue; urine too yellow; halitosis.

Treatment: Needle: 1/8 inch.
Moxa: 3 times, 1/4 rice grain size.

Stimulus: Painful feeling in the upper lip.

30.8 **Y'n Jiao** *gum crossing* **GV-28**

Location: In the upper tip of the frenulum superioris.

Effects: Sores; ringworm on the face of children; excessive weeping; white film over the eyes; nose blocked; nasal polyps; melancholia in chest; jaundice; halitosis.

Treatment: Needle: 1/8 inch.
No Moxa.

Stimulus: Lightly painful.

Section 31 **Lung Meridian**

31.1 **Yun Men** *cloud door* **LU-2**

Location: 1 and 3/8 divisions above LU-1; 6 divisions starting from between first and second ribs lateral to the Conception Vessel meridian.

Effects: Coldness in the four limbs because of the flu; bouts of coughing; shortness of breath; feeling of oppression and pain on the chest; fullness of the chest; pain on the back and shoulders; cannot raise arms; tonsillitis; acne; melancholia in chest.

Treatment: **No Needle**.
Moxa: 5 times.
Needle here will damage the arms making it difficult to raise them.

Stimulus: Radiating to the center of the chest.

31.2 **Tian Fu** *heavenly mansion* **LU-3**

Location: 6 divisions above the elbow crease slanting up between the two muscles.

Effects: Epistaxis; after apoplexy, patient crying and laughing or talking nonsense; depression; dizziness in the eyes; dimness of vision; bronchitis.

Treatment: Needle: 1/4 to 1/2 inch.
No Moxa.

Stimulus: Down to the wrist.

31.3 **Xia Bai** *chivalry white* **LU-4**

Location: 5 divisions above the elbow crease slanting up between two muscles.

Effects: Pain on the chest; cardiac pain; nausea; melancholia.

Treatment: Needle: 1/4 to 1/2 inch.
Moxa: 5 times.

Stimulus: Down to the wrist.

31.4 **Kung Tsui** *supreme hole* **LU-6**

Location: 5 divisions below LU-5, slanting down toward the radial bone on a muscle cleft.

Effects: High fever without perspiration; sore throat; loss of voice; hemoptysis; tonsillitis; headache; pain on the arm, difficult to bend, stretch or raise up; fingers cannot clench.

Treatment: Needle: 1/4 inch or a little more.
Moxa: 5 times.

Stimulus: Down to the hand.

31.5 **Yu Ji** *fish border* **LU-10**

Location: On the palmar surface, at the anterior edge of the first metacarpal, behind the joint. Bend the thumb to find the joint.

Effects: Cold sensations from excessive drinking; coughing; yellow coating of the tongue; high fever with headache; flu without perspiration; chest and back painful; dizziness of the eyes; melancholia; shortness of breath; stomach pains with anorexia; dryness of the throat; pain on the arm; incontinence; urination from coughing; hemoptysis; frightened condition; breast abscess; pain on palm.

Treatment: Needle: 1/8 to 1/4 inch.
No Moxa.

Stimulus: Down to the thumb causing the local muscles to jump.

Section 32 **Heart Meridian**

32.1 **Ji Chuan** *extreme spring* **HT-1**

Location: Top center of the armpit, by palpation with the fingers the reaction should be felt down to the little finger.

Effects: Pain in chest and ribs; full feeling in chest; cardiac pain; nausea; moral depression; jaundice in eyes; forearm cold, difficult to raise up; weak eyesight; body odor.

Treatment: Needle: 1/4 to 1/2 inch.
Moxa: 7 times.

Stimulus: Down the arm and small finger.

32.2 **Ching Ling** *green spirit* **HT-2**

Location: 3 divisions above the tip of the elbow in the cleft of the muscles, on the medial side of the arm.

Effects: Jaundiced eyes; headache; chills; intercostal pain; inability to raise arms; cannot wear clothes.

Treatment: **No Needle**.
Moxa 3 to 7 times.

Stimulus: Down to the small finger.

Section 33 **Pericardium Meridian**

33.1 **Tian Chi** *heavenly pond* **PC-1**

Location: One division lateral to the nipple between two ribs, which puts the point a little higher than the nipple.

Effects: Noises from breathing; full feeling in chest; fever without perspiration; headache; difficulty raising the four limbs; swelling under the armpit; adenitis; insufficient lactation; mammary pain; chi rushing up; fever and chills similar to malaria; foggy vision; pain on the arm.

Treatment: Needle: 1/4 inch.
Moxa: 3 times.

Stimulus: Up the chest and across to the armpit.

33.2 **Tian Chuan** *heavenly spring* **PC-2**

Location: Seven divisions above PC-3 on the inside of the arm.

Effects: Foggy vision; fear of cold winds; cardiac pain; full feeling in the chest; coughing; pain radiating from the chest to the back; pain along the inside of the arm.

Treatment: Needle: 1/4 to 1/2 inch.
Moxa: 3 times.

Stimulus: Down to the elbow crease.

Section 34 **Large Intestine Meridian**

34.1 **Erh Jien** *second interval* **LI-2**

Location: Just distal to the first metacarpal joint of the pointing finger, at the meeting of the yin and yang skins.

Effects: Epistaxis; jaundice; toothache; throat numb; tonsillitis; spasm of esophagus; vision confused; pain on shoulder and arm; swollen jaw; facial palsy; dryness of the mouth; overcooling conditions with water retention.

Treatment: Needle: 1/8 to 1/4 inch.
Moxa: 3 times.

Stimulus: Down the finger.

34.2 **San Jian** *third interval* **LI-3**

Location: Just proximal to the first metacarpal joint of the pointing finger, under the metacarpal bone.

Effects: Numb throat; feeling of something stuck in the throat; tonsillitis; eye pain; itching on eyelids; dyspnea; mouth and lips dry; tongue extended, difficult to retract; diarrhea; excessive mucus in the throat causing coughing; toothache; flu with hot sensations; overcooling conditions with water retention.

Treatment: Needle: 1/4 inch.
Moxa: 3 times.

Stimulus: Around the joint and out to the finger.

34.3 **Pian Lih** *inclined passage* **LI-6**

Location: 3 divisions above the wrist (LI-5) at the outer edge of the radial bone on the posterior external surface of the forearm.

Effects: Pain in shoulder and elbow; dimness of vision; fever; madness; mad speech; throat dry and numb; tonsillitis; epistaxis; deafness; toothache; retention of urine.

Treatment: Needle: 1/4 to 1/3 inch.
Moxa 3 to 5 times.

Stimulus: Reaction down the hand.

34.4 **Wen Liu** *warm current* **LI-7**

Location: 3 divisions above LI-6, along the outer edge of the radial bone, following the Large Intestine line up to the elbow.

Effects: Borborygmi from intestines; four limbs swollen; throat numb; insanity; sees "devils;" swollen tongue; glossitis; belching; fever and headache; cannot retract tongue; tonsillitis.

Treatment: Needle: 1/4 to 1/2 inch.
Moxa: 3 to 5 times.

Stimulus: Down to the index finger.

34.5 **Xia Lian** *lower screen* **LI-8**

Location: 2 divisions above LI-7 on the top of the muscle.

Effects: Tuberculosis with diarrhea; full feeling in lower abdomen; blood in urine; hematuria; crazy speech; paralysis of one side of the body; numbness; pale face; sharp pains in the abdomen, like a knife twisting inside; painful abdomen, groin, umbilical region; running around madly; dyspnea; chapped lips; clear saliva dribbling from mouth; carbuncle on breast.

Treatment: Needle: 1/4 to 1/2 inch.
Moxa: 3 to 5 times.

Stimulus: Felt down to the hand.

34.6 **Shang Lian** *upper screen* **LI-9**

Location: One division above LI-8; 3 divisions below LI-11.

Effects: Borborygmi; difficult urination; urine icteric or red; pain on chest; hemiplegia; cold sensations in the bones and marrow; numbness in the four limbs; dyspnea; gas in intestines; overcooling headache.

Treatment: Needle: 1/4 to 1/2 inch.
Moxa: 5 times.

Stimulus: Down to the hand.

34.7 **Joou Liao** *elbow bone* **LI-12**

Location: One division slanting outwards from LI-11 in the corner of the humerus and radial bone; to locate this point, put the hand on the chest and bend the arm.

Effects: Excessive sleep; elbow pain/numbness; arm pain, unable to raise the arm; arm cramping or numb.

Treatment: Needle: 1/4 to 1/2 inch.
Moxa: 3 to 5 times.

Stimulus: Around the elbow.

34.8 **Tian Ding** *heavenly vessel* **LI-17**

Location: Starting at the tip of the Adams apple (CV-23), go lateral to the outer edge of the larynx (this is ST-9); then go down one division to the outer edge of the thyroid; this is the point.

Effects: Sudden muteness; numb, swollen throat with dyspnea; cannot swallow; wheezing.

Treatment: Needle: 3/8 inch.
Moxa: 3 times.

Stimulus: Up to the neck and down to the chest.

34.9 **Fu Tu** *support and rush* **LI-18**

Location: One division (the foreneck is divided into 3 divisions) above LI-17 slanting up the outer edge of the thyroid gland.

Effects: Shortness of breath; sounds with breathing; sudden muteness; coughing up a lot of mucus.

Treatment: Needle: 1/4 inch.
Moxa: 3 times.

Stimulus: Up to the temple, down to the chest.

34.10 **Ho Liao** *grain bone* **LI-19**

Location: About one-half eye division lateral to GV-26 (in the center of the philtrum) on the line of the outer edge of the nostril.

Effects: Nose obstructed; nasal catarrh; mouth paralyzed; epistaxis; nasal polyps; anosmia; shock.

Treatment: Needle: 1/8 inch or a little deeper.
No Moxa.

Stimulus: Strong painful stimulus of the lip provoking patient to tears.

Section 35 **Triple Warmer Meridian**

35.1 **Hui Jung** *meeting ancestor* **TW-7**

Location: 3 divisions above the wrist on the back of the forearm, one-half division lateral to TW-6 at the edge of the ulnar bone.

Effects: Deafness; epilepsy; skin and flesh painful.

Treatment: **No Needle** according to the old books.
Moxa: 3 times.

Stimulus: Down to the fingers.

35.2 **San Yang Lo** *3 yang binders* **TW-8**

Location: 4 divisions up from the middle of the wrist (TW-4) in beween the ulnar and radial bones.

Effects: Acute muteness; deafness; excessive sleeping; patient too tired to move arms, legs and torso.

Treatment: **No Needle**.
Moxa: 3 to 7 times.

Stimulus: Down to the hand.

35.3 **Si Du** *four gutters* **TW-9**

Location: 5 divisions below the elbow; 3 divisions above TW-8, slanting up between the two muscles.

Effects: Acute deafness; lower jaw toothache.

Treatment: Needle: 1/2 inch.
Moxa: 5 to 7 times.

Stimulus: Down to the wrist.

35.4 **Tian Jing** *heavenly well* **TW-10**

Location: Located on the posterior surface of the arm; one division above the point of the elbow in the depression between the bone and the muscle. To locate this point, bend the elbow 90 degrees.

Effects: Pain on the chest; coughing with short breaths; speech difficult; spitting up pus; anorexia; epistaxis; cold sensations; high temperature; cannot lie down; deafness; throat swollen or numb; excessive perspiration; outer corners of the eyes red and painful; elbow/arm pain; unable to grasp objects; excessive sleeping; lumbago; neck pain with chills; depressed; worried spirit; beri-beri.

Treatment: Needle: 1/2 inch.
Moxa: 3 to 5 times.

Stimulus: Around the elbow, slightly up the arm.

35.5 **Ching Leng Yuan** *pure cold abyss* **TW-11**

Location: One division straight up from TW-10; in a depression between the bone and the muscle.

Effects: Pain on arm and/or shoulder; cannot raise arm up; cannot bear to wear clothes.

Treatment: Needle: 1/4 inch.
Moxa: 3 times.

Stimulus: Slightly up and down from the point.

35.6 **Hsiao Leh** *thawing Leh River* **TW-12**

Location: 4 divisions above TW-11 in the center of the posterior surface of the arm.

Effects: Arms/back swollen and painful; neck swollen and painful; headache; madness.

Treatment: Needle: 1/4 to 1/2 inch.
Moxa: 3 times.

Stimulus: Felt locally.

35.7 **Nao Hui** *arm meeting* **TW-13**

Location: 2 divisions straight up from TW-12.

Effects: Arm painful and sore, difficult to raise; shoulder swollen and painful with the pain spreading to the scapula region; neck tumors; goiters.

Treatment: Needle: 1/4 to 1/2 inch.
Moxa: 5 times.

Stimulus: Down to the elbow.

35.8 **Jian Liao** *shoulder bone* **TW-14**

Location: At the same level as LI-15, towards the back of the shoulder two finger divisions, in a depression below the bone.

Effects: Pain in shoulder and arm; patient cannot raise up the arm.

Treatment: Needle: 1/2 inch.
Moxa 3 to 5 times.

Stimulus: Felt locally and a little down the arm.

35.9 **Tian Liao** *heavenly bone* **TW-15**

Location: 5 divisions lateral to GV-14.

Effects: Melancholia; pain/soreness of the shoulder; absence of perspiration; full feeling in the chest; neck stiffness.

Treatment: Needle: 1/2 inch.
Moxa: 3 times.

Stimulus: Up to the neck, down to the shoulder.

35.10 **Tin Yau** *window of heaven* **TW-16**

Location: Go one division below GB-20 and then lateral 1/2 division.

Effects: Sudden deafness; partial deafness; dim vision; lively dreams; face swollen, pale, and yellow; neck stiff, cannot turn; eyes painful.

Treatment: Needle: 1/2 to 3/4 inch.
No Moxa.
Moxa here will cause the patient's face to swell, closing the eyes.

Stimulus: Up to the temple and down the back of the neck.

35.11 **Chi Mo** *madness pulse* **TW-18**

Location: One divisions above TW-17 close to the edge of the ear, in a small vertical cleft formed under the bone on the level of GB-2.

Effects: Tinnitus; cramping in children; convulsions; vomiting; diarrhea; terror; excessive yellow matter in the eyes.

Treatment: Needle: 1/16 to 1/8 inch.
Moxa: 3 times.

Stimulus: Reaction felt towards the back of the head, part to the back of the ear.

35.12 **Lu Xi** *skull rest* **TW-19**

Location: 1 and 1/2 divisions above TW-18; which is also approximately 3/5 of the vertical distance between TW-17 and TW-20, behind the earlobe at the horizontal cleft at the level of TW-21.

Effects: Tinnitus; dyspnea; vomiting saliva in children; epilepsy; pain spreading from the chest to the sides of the body; headache with high temperature; ear swollen; middle ear inflamed.

Treatment: Needle: 1/12 inch.
Moxa: 3 times.

Stimulus: Reaction down to the back of the head and locally.

Note: Do not bleed this point, it would kill the patient.

35.13 **Jiao Sin** *angle of the ear* **TW-20**

Location: At the apex of the ear on the hairline in a vertical cleft.

Effects: Film on the eyes; gums swollen; lips stiff; difficulty chewing; headache and neck stiff.

Treatment: Needle: 1/12 to 1/8 inch.
Moxa: 3 times.

Stimulus: Reaction up the side of the head towards the temples, and to the back of the head.

35.14 **Ho Liao** *harmony bone* **TW-22**

Location: 1/2 division above TW-21 and 1/4 division towards the face at the horizontal cleft. There is a pulse here.

Effects: Headaches; jaw stiff; neck swollen; tinnitus; running nose; patient is afraid to expose their face to the cold; tip of the nose swollen; facial spasm.

Treatment: Needle: 1/4 inch.
Moxa: 3 times.

Stimulus: Up the side of the head and towards the temples.

Section 36 **Small Intestine Meridian**

36.1 **Chien Ku** *front valley* **SI-2**

Location: On the outside edge of the hand, at the meeting of the yin and yang skin, just distal to the metacarpophalangeal joint of the little finger.

Effects: High temperature without perspiration; malaria; tinnitus; neck swollen; throat numb; swollen jaw with pain radiating to behind the ear; coughing; hematemesis; epistaxis; arm pain, cannot elevate; no lactation after childbirth.

Treatment: Needle: 1/8 inch.
Moxa: 1 to 3 times.

Stimulus: Around the joint, down to the small finger.

36.2 **Yang Lao** *supporting the old* **SI-6**

Location: Just proximal to the head of the ulnar bone. There is a big cleft when the wrist is bent; this is the point, behind the eminence of the round bone.

Effects: Sore and painful shoulder and upper arm (that is, pain as if the arm were broken), stiff as if someone was pulling the arm out of its socket; dim vision.

Treatment: Needle: 1/4 inch.
Moxa: 3 times.

Stimulus: Reaction up the ulnar bone, down to the wrist.

36.3 **Jie Jeng** *support straight* **SI-7**

Location: 5 divisions above the wrist crease; on the inner edge of the ulnar bone.

Effects: Patient frightened, worried, insane; four limbs weak; arm cramped, difficult to stretch; pains in all fingers, cannot clench hand; neck sores; thirst; neck stiff; small neck tumor.

Treatment: Needle: 1/4 inch.
Moxa: 3 to 5 times.

Stimulus: Up and down from the point several inches.

36.4 **Jian Jieng** *shoulder chastity* **SI-9**

Location: Approximately 7 divisions lateral to GV-11, directly above the posterior axillary fold.

Effects: Patient with the flu; high temperature and chills; tinnitus; deafness; hot sensations on the shoulder above the clavicle; pain and/or numbness of arms, cannot elevate.

Treatment: Needle: 1/2 inch.
Moxa: 3 to 5 times.

Stimulus: Up to shoulder area and also locally.

36.5 **Nau Yu** *shoulder blade yu* **SI-10**

Location: 7 divisions lateral to GV-12.

Effects: Arms sore and weak; unable to raise arm; hot and cold feelings; neck swollen and painful.

Treatment: Needle: 1/2 inch.
Moxa: 3 to 5 times.

Stimulus: Felt locally.

36.6 **Tien Jung** *heavenly ancestor* **SI-11**

Location: 5 divisions lateral to the depession under the fourth thoracic vertebra.

Effects: Arms and shoulders sore and painful; pain on outer side of the elbow; jaw swollen.

Treatment: Needle: 1/4 to 1/2 inch.
Moxa: 3 times.

Stimulus: Up and down the edge of the scapula.

36.7 **Bin Feng** *facing the wind* **SI-12**

Location: Between GV-13 and GV-14 (the 1st thoracic bone), lateral 5 divisions, directly above SI-11.

Effects: Shoulder and arm neuralgia and numbness; cannot elevate arm.

Treatment: Needle: 1/4 to 1/2 inch.
Moxa: 5 times.

Stimulus: Felt up to the neck and shoulder.

36.8 **Chu Yuan** *crooked wall* **SI-13**

Location: 3 and 1/2 divisions lateral to a point under the second thoracic vertebrae.

Effects: Neuralgia/numbness of the shoulder/arm; shoulder hot; patient unable to embrace.

Treatment: Needle: 1/2 inch or a little deeper.
Moxa: 3 to 5 times.

Stimulus: Up to the neck.

36.9 **Jian Wai Yu**

outside of the shoulder yu **SI-14**

Location: 2 and 1/2 divisions lateral to the midpoint between the second and third thoracic vertebrae.

Effects: Spasm; muscle pain and neuralgia of the shoulder/arm; cold feelings starting at the shoulder and spreading to the elbow.

Treatment: Needle: 1/4 to 1/2 inch.
Moxa: 3 times.

Stimulus: Lateral to the upper back and shoulder.

36.10 **Jian Jung Yu** *middle of the shoulder yu* **SI-15**

Location: 2 divisions lateral to GV-14.

Effects: Coughing; shortness of breath; hemoptysis; cold and hot sensation on the back; dim vision.

Treatment: Needle: 1/4 inch.
Moxa: 5 to 10 times.

Stimulus: Lateral to the top of the shoulder.

36.11 **Tian Chang** *heavenly window* **SI-16**

Location: 1 eye division behind LI-18, and a little higher.

Effects: Anal fistula; pain on the neck and shoulder; neck stiff; cannot turn head; deafness; jaw swollen; tonsillitis; acute muteness following a stroke.

Treatment: Needle: 1/4 to 1/2 inch.
Moxa: 3 times.

Stimulus: Up the neck and down the shoulder.

36.12 **Tien Yung** *heavenly appearance* **SI-17**

Location: At the same level as ST-6 behind the jawbone 1/8 inch.

Effects: Throat numb; feelings of something being caught in the pharynx; lumps or abscess on the neck; patient cannot speak or turn their neck; chest painful; full breathing difficult; vomiting excess saliva; tinnitus; deafness.

Treatment: Needle: 1/4 inch.
Moxa: 3 times.

Stimulus: Down the neck and up to the ear.

36.13 **Chuan Liao** *cheekbone hole* **SI-18**

Location: In the hollow below the middle of the cheekbone.

Effects: Facial paralysis; trigeminal neuralgia; red face; eyes jaundiced; eye twitch; jaw swollen without toothache.

Treatment: Needle: 1/4 inch.
No Moxa.

Stimulus: Felt going towards the nose and mouth.

Section 37 **Kidney Meridian**

37.1 **Shui Chuan** *water spring* **KI-5**

Location: One division directly below KI-3.

Effects: Blurred vision; irregular menstruation; melancholia in chest and abdominal pains during menstruation; prolapse of uterus; abdominal pain; frequent micturition.

Treatment: Needle: 1/4 inch.
Moxa: 3 to 5 times.

Stimulus: Around the heel.

37.2 **Chu Bin** *building guests* **KI-9**

Location: 5 divisions above the medial malleolus, 3 divisions directly above KI-7, between two muscles.

Effects: Madness; crazy talking; scolding; tongue stretched out; vomiting saliva; hernia in a child; calves painful.

Treatment: Needle: 1/4 to 1/2 inch.
Moxa: 5 times.

Stimulus: Up the calf, down to the foot.

37.3 **Yin Gu** *yin valley* **KI-10**

Location: In between BL-54 and LV-8 at the same level as BL-54, between the two tendons at the medial edge of the inner knee crease.

Effects: Sharp pains in the knee; knee cannot be bent or stretched; tongue hanging out and patient dribbling saliva; dysuria; pain felt in urethra just before urination; impotence; pain on the inner side of the thigh; spotting between periods; abdomen swollen and breathing difficult; man's stomach swollen similar to dropsy and/or woman's stomach swollen as in pregnancy, but from worms, poison, etc.

Treatment: Needle: 1/2 inch.
Moxa: 3 times.

Stimulus: Goes down to the foot.

37.4 **Heng Gu** *transverse bone (pubis)* **KI-11**

Location: 1/2 division lateral to CV-2, at the edge of the pubic bone.

Effects: Gonorrhea; anuria; lower abdomen swollen; all yin organs weak; loss of semen; eyes red/painful starting from the inner canthus.

Treatment: **No Needle.**
Moxa: 3 times.

Stimulus: Reaction a little down to the scrotum and across the pubic bone.

37.5 **Da Heh** *big brightness* **KI-12**

Location: One division above KI-11, 1/2 division lateral to CV-3.

Effects: Gas moving up and down in the abdomen causing lower back pain; chronic diarrhea; irregular menses; eyes red/painful starting from inner canthus; spermatorrhea; pain in the penis; vaginal discharge.

Treatment: Needle: 1/4 to 1/2 inch.
Moxa: 3 times.

Stimulus: Local.

37.6 **Chi Hsueh** *chi hole* **KI-13**

Location: 1/2 division lateral to CV-4.

Effects: Gas in the abdomen running up and down causing back pain; chronic diarrhea; eyes red/painful starting at inner canthus; irregular menses.

Treatment: Needle: 1/2 to 3/4 inch.
Moxa: 3 times.

Stimulus: Local.

37.7 **Szi Men** *four full* **KI-14**

Location: 1/2 division lateral to CV-5.

Effects: Hernia below the navel; abundant stools; cutting pains below the navel; shivering without cold; eyes red/painful from inner canthus; irregular periods; menorrhalgia; gas running around in abdomen; woman has difficulty conceiving.

Treatment: Needle: 1/4 to 1/2 inch.
Moxa: 3 times.

Stimulus: Local.

37.8 **Jung Ju** *middle injection* **KI-15**

Location: 1/2 division lateral to CV-7.

Effects: Hot sensations in the lower abdomen; constipation; irregular menses; inner canthus red/painful.

Treatment: Needle: 1/4 inch or a little more.
Moxa: 5 times.

Stimulus: Local.

37.9 **Fong Yu** *vital yu* **KI-16**

Location: 1/2 division lateral to the center of the umbilicus (CV-8).

Effects: Cutting pains in the abdomen; constipation; diarrhea; abdomen swollen and full; chilled sensations below chest; inner canthus red/painful.

Treatment: Needle: 1/2 to 3/4 inch.
Moxa: 5 times.

Stimulus: Local.

37.10 **Shang Chu** *merchant's tune* **KI-17**

Location: 1/2 division lateral to CV-10.

Effects: Abdomen painful; cutting pains when abdomen is full; anorexia; eye painful starting at inner canthus.

Treatment: Needle: 1/2 to 3/4 inch.
Moxa: 5 times.

Stimulus: Local.

37.11 **Shi Guan** *stone gate* **KI-18**

Location: 1/2 division lateral to CV-11.

Effects: Belching; gastric pain; constipation; urine deep yellow; epigastrium swollen; stiffness of the spine; frequent spitting; eyes red/painful from inner canthus; female sterility; lower abdomen pain felt up to the chest (in females only).

Treatment: Needle: 1/2 to 3/4 inch.
Moxa: 3 to 5 times.

Stimulus: Local.

37.12 **Yin Du** *ghost's capital* **KI-19**

Location: 1/2 division lateral to CV-12.

Effects: Body chills/fevers; melancholia under the chest area; borborygmi; full feeling in lungs; sides of the body hot/painful; inner canthus red/painful.

Treatment: Needle: 1/2 to 1 inch.
Moxa: 3 times.

Stimulus: Local.

37.13 **Tung Gu** *penetrating valley, abdomen* **KI-20**

Location 1/2 division lateral to CV-13.

Effects: Paralysis of the face by yawning; vomiting after eating; sudden acute muteness; water stagnating in stomach; indigestion; full feelings under the chest; insanity; inner canthus red/painful.

Treatment: Needle: 1/2 to 3/4 inch.
Moxa: 5 times.

Stimulus: Local.

37.14 **You Men** *gate of hades* **KI-21**

Location: 1/2 division lateral to CV-14.

Effects: Full feeling in the lower abdomen; vomiting with saliva/phlegm; frequent spitting; melancholia in chest; anorexia; forgetfulness; diarrhea with blood and pus, in female; pains in the chest; belching; diarrhea; difficulty eating; inner canthus red/painful.

Treatment: Needle: 1/2 inch.
Moxa: 5 times.

Stimulus: Local.

37.15 **Bu Long** *walking corridor* **KI-22**

Location: 2 divisions lateral to CV-16.

Effects: Chest and ribs full; dyspnea; coughing; nose blocked; anorexia; pain on chest; cannot raise arms.

Treatment: Needle: 1/4 inch.
Moxa: 5 times.

Stimulus: Up and down the chest from the point.

37.16 **Shen Feng** *spirit seal* **KI-23**

Location: 2 divisions lateral to CV-17.

Effects: Coughing; chest full; patient cannot breathe; carbuncle/tumor on the breast; chills and fevers; anorexia.

Treatment: Needle: 1/4 inch.
Moxa: 5 times.

Stimulus: Up and down from the point.

37.17 **Ling Shu** *spirit market* **KI-24**

Location: 2 divisions lateral to CV-18.

Effects: Chest full and painful; incessant coughing; dyspnea; bronchitis; vomiting; chest melancholia; stuffed nose; anosmia; anorexia; cramping on the chest; carbuncle on the breast; inflammation of the mammary gland.

Treatment: Needle: 1/4 inch.
Moxa: 5 times.

Stimulus: Up and down from the point.

37.18 **Shen Tsang** *spirit store* **KI-25**

Location: 2 divisions lateral to CV-19.

Effects: Chest and ribs full; coughing and dyspnea; bronchitis; vomiting; anorexia; intercostal neuralgia; pulmonary congestion.

Treatment: Needle: 1/4 inch.
Moxa: 5 times.

Stimulus: Up and down from the point.

37.19 **Yu Jung** *amidst elegance* **KI-26**

Location: 2 divisions lateral to CV-20.

Effects: Coughing; dyspnea; full feeling in chest and sides of body; excessive saliva/spitting; intercostal neuralgia; pleurisy; vomiting; anorexia.

Treatment: Needle: 1/4 inch.
Moxa: 5 times.

Stimulus: To both sides of point and going up.

37.20 **Yu Fu** *yu mansion* **KI-27**

Location: 2 divisions lateral to CV-21.

Effects: Coughing; chest full; cannot breathe; chest painful; chronic asthma (moxa 7 times); vomiting; anorexia.

Treatment: Needle: 1/4 inch.
Moxa: 5 times.

Stimulus: To both sides of the point and up to the clavicle.

Section 38 **Spleen Meridian**

38.1 **Tai Bai** *supreme whiteness* **SP-3**

Location: On the medial side of the distal end of the metatarsal bone of the big toe, just proximal to the joint, where the yin and yang skin meet.

Effects: Fever; melancholia on chest; swollen abdomen; indigestion; vomiting; diarrhea with pus and blood; back pain associated with constipation; vomiting, diarrhea and abdominal pain; borborygmi; pain in the knee; spasm of the legs; body heavy, with painful joints; pain on chest and stomach; pain under the chest with low blood pressure.

Treatment: Needle: 1/4 inch.
Moxa: 3 times.

Stimulus: Reaction to the end of the big toe.

38.2 **Lou Gu** *leaky valley* **SP-7**

Location: 6 divisions proximal to the upper edge of the medial malleolus, almost directly above SP-6, one-half division behind the tibia bone.

Effects: Borborygmi; indigestion; flatulence; patient eats a lot but does not gain weight; dysuria; numbness of knee/leg with difficulty walking.

Treatment: Needle: 1/2 inch.
No Moxa.

Stimulus: Down to the ankle.

38.3 **De Jee** *earth secret* **SP-8**

Location: 3 divisions directly below SP-9; between two muscles.

Effects: Back pains; difficulty bending/straightening; the abdomen and the sides of the body painful; dropsy; anorexia; dysuria; sterility in males; woman with distended stomach (touching it creates a wave); pain on the inner thigh/knee.

Treatment: Needle: 1/2 inch.
Moxa: 3 times.

Stimulus: Up to the knee; down the calf.

38.4 **Jee Men** *basket door* **SP-11**

Location: 6 divisions directly above SP-10; in between two muscles.

Effects: Gonorrhea in males; anuria; incontinence of urine; inguinal adenitis.

Treatment: Needle: 1/2 inch.
Moxa: 3 times.

Stimulus: Up and down from the point.

38.5 **Chung Men** *rushing door* **SP-12**

Location: 3 and 1/2 divisions lateral to CV-2.

Effects: Cold sensations in the abdomen; abdomen distended; pain in abdomen; excessive secretion on the part of the female during sexual intercourse; pregnant woman with difficulty breathing and "pulling down" feelings in chest; no lactation.

Treatment: Needle: 1/4 inch.
Moxa: 7 times.

Stimulus: Local.

38.6 **Fu Sheh** *mansion cottage* **SP-13**

Location: 3/4 of a division above SP-12; 4 divisions lateral to the Conception Vessel line.

Effects: Hernia; pain in sides radiating to chest; indigestion; abdomen painful; cholera.

Treatment: Needle: 1/4 inch.
Moxa: 5 times.

Stimulus: Down to the thigh.

38.7 **Fu Jie** *abdomen knot* **SP-14**

Location: 4 divisions lateral to the point midway between CV-6 and CV-7.

Effects: Overcooling in the abdomen; patient cries too easily; four limbs immobile; excessive perspiration; diarrhea.

Treatment: Needle: 1/2 to 3/4 inch.
Moxa: 5 times.

Stimulus: Reaction felt down the Spleen line on the lower abdomen.

38.8 **Da Heng** *big horizontal* **SP-15**

Location: 4 divisions lateral to the center of the umbilicus.

Effects: Overcooling in the abdomen; chi felt rising up in the chest; difficulty moving the four limbs; patient always sad.

Treatment: Needle: 1/4 to 1/2 inch.
Moxa: 3 to 5 times.

Stimulus: Reaction felt down the Spleen line on the lower abdomen.

38.9 **Fu Ai** *abdomen sorrow* **SP-16**

Location: 4 divisions lateral to CV-11.

Effects: Overcooling in abdomen; indigestion; blood and/or pus in the stool.

Treatment: Needle: 1/4 to 1/2 inch.
Moxa: 3 to 5 times.

Stimulus: Local.

38.10 **Shi Dou** *food drain* **SP-17**

Location: 2 divisions lateral to ST-18 and at the same intercostal space.

Effects: Chest and sides of ribs have a full feeling; borborygmi in diaphragm area; sounds of water moving around the diaphragm area; pain in diaphragm.

Treatment: Needle: 1/4 inch.
Moxa: 5 times.

Stimulus: Lateral to both sides of the point.

Note: Raise patient's arms to locate the point above.

38.11 **Tian Xi** *heavenly stream* **SP-18**

Location: 6 divisions lateral to a point midway between CV-17 and CV-18; between two ribs.

Effects: Chest full with a full feeling and pain; coughing; chi felt rushing up the chest; wheezing from bronchi; swollen breasts; carbuncle on the breasts.

Treatment: Needle: 1/4 inch or a little more.
Moxa: 5 times.

Stimulus: Felt inward to the breast.

Note: To locate the point above, the patient should lie down.

38.12 **Shung Shiang** *chest village* **SP-19**

Location: 6 divisions lateral to a point midway between CV-18 and CV-19.

Effects: Chest and ribs feel full; pain felt from chest to back; difficulty lying down, turning the body from side to side.

Treatment: Needle: 1/4 inch or a little more.
Moxa: 5 times.

Stimulus: Felt across the chest between the two rib bones.

38.13 **Jou Yung** *encircling glory* **SP-20**

Location: 6 divisions lateral to a point midway between CV-19 and CV-20.

Effects: Chest, ribs and abdomen distended, cannot raise up, cannot bend, and feels full; patient cannot eat, but likes to drink water; coughing; spitting; belching, with pus; lust.

Treatment: Needle: 1/4 inch or a little more.
Moxa: 5 times.

Stimulus: Felt locally.

38.14 **Da Bao** *big enveloping* **SP-21**

Location: 8 divisions lateral to CV-14, 4 divisions lateral to LV-14.

Effects: Dyspnea with chest pain; body overheating; all joints painful (needle); body overcooling and with all joints seeming slightly disjointed; patient lacks energy (moxa).

Treatment: Needle: 1/4 inch.
Moxa: 3 to 5 times.

Stimulus: Felt to both sides of the point.

Section 39 **Liver Meridian**

39.1 **Li Kou** *insect ditch* **LV-5**

Location: 5 divisions above the upper edge of the medial malleolus, behind the border of the tibia.

Effects: Violent pain in the lower abdomen; dysuria; patient frightened, or unhappy; discomfort in area of pharynx; back cramped; difficult for patient to get up, or bend; gas stagnant in the lower abdomen, like a stone; cold, sore sensations in the tibia; difficulty moving the lower leg; vaginal discharge; irregular period; pain in the testicles; itching in the scrotum.

Treatment: Needle: 1/4 to 1/2 inch.
Moxa: 3 times.

Stimulus: Up to the knee; down to the ankle.

39.2 **Jung Du** *middle capital* **LV-6**

Location: 7 divisions above the upper edge of the medial malleolus.

Effects: Lower abdominal pain; patient cannot walk/stand; cold sensations in the tibia; menorrhagia after childbirth.

Treatment: Needle: 1/4 to 1/2 inch.
Moxa: 5 times.

Stimulus: Several inches up and down from the point.

39.3 **Yin Bao** *yin wrapping* **LV-9**

Location: 4 divisions above the back knee crease; in the middle of the inner thigh, between two muscles.

Effects: Pain from the base of the spine radiating to the lower abdomen; dysuria; bedwetting; irregular menses.

Treatment: Needle: 1/2 to 3/4 inch.
Moxa: 3 to 5 times.

Stimulus: Up to the groin, down to the knee.

39.4 **Wu Li** *(foot) 5 mile* **LV-10**

Location: 3 divisions below ST-30, lateral to the big tendon. One division below LV-11.

Effects: Full feelings in the lower abdomen; hot sensations; dysuria; excessive sleeping; patient cannot raise the four limbs.

Treatment: Needle: 1/2 inch.
Moxa: 5 times.

Stimulus: Felt several inches down the inner side of the thigh.

39.5 **Ji Mai** *quick pulse* **LV-12**

Location: 1 division directly below ST-30 on top of the pubic bone.

Effects: Pain of penis or scrotum.

Treatment: **No Needle.**
Moxa: 5 times.

Stimulus: A little down the scrotum.

Section 40 **Stomach Meridian**

40.1 **Cheng Chi** *receive tears* **ST-1**

Location: 1/2 inch directly below the eyelid, with the eyes looking straight ahead.

Effects: Eyes with cold sensations and tears; eyes locked looking up; itching in eyes; dim vision; night blindness; shaking of the eyeball; paralysis of the face; difficult to speak; face twisted; eyes red and painful; tinnitus; deafness.

Treatment: According to the old book:
No Needle.
Moxa: 3 times.
A needle here would turn the whole eye black.
Another book says to needle: 3/8 inch. It also says no moxa; moxa here will cause the eye to swell as big as a fist and will cause nasal polyps to expand to the size of a peach; after 30 days the eye will be blind.
The third book says: No Needle, No Moxa.

40.2 **Si Bai** *four whites* **ST-2**

Location: 1 inch directly below the eyelid with eyes looking straight ahead.

Effects: Headache; dizziness in the eye; eyes red/painful; dim vision; eyes itching; eyes have vision as if smoke is inside the eye; facial paralysis and muteness.

Treatment: Needle: 1/8 to 1/4 inch.
No Moxa.
No Deep Needle; if too deep the eye will turn black.

Stimulus: Around the lower orbital.

40.3 **Ju Liao** *great bone* **ST-3**

Location: At the same level as the inferior border of the nose, directly below the middle of the eye.

Effects: Facial spasm; lips/jaws swollen/painful; facial paralysis; myopia; a white spot in the iris, covering the pupil; abscess of the nose; beri-beri; knee swollen; cataract.

Treatment: Needle: 1/4 inch.
Moxa: 7 times.

Stimulus: Up the cheek, down to the lips.

40.4 **Da Ying** *big welcome* **ST-5**

Location: One eye division in front of the angle of the jaw bone, in a vertical hollow in the jawbone.

Effects: After a stroke, mouth closed shut; lips trembling; jaw swollen, toothache; pain in the neck with chills and fever; scrofula; facial paralysis; tongue stiff; face swollen; eye pain, cannot open.

Treatment: Needle: 1/4 inch.
Moxa: 3 times. There is a pulse here.

Stimulus: Up to the jaw, down to the chin.

40.5 **Shia Guan** *lower gate* **ST-7**

Location: One eye division in front of SI-19, in the hollow under the cheek bone. Close the mouth and there is a hollow at this point. When the mouth is opened wide, a bone moves in front of the point.

Effects: Inflammation of the middle ear; facial paralysis; loosening of the jaw; gums swollen.

Treatment: Needle: 1/4 inch, pull out needle immediately after obtaining the stimulus; do not leave the needle in the point.
No Moxa.

Stimulus: Up to the temple, down the cheek bone.

40.6 **Yen Ying** *man welcome* **ST-9**

Location: 1 and 1/2 divisions lateral to the center of the Adam's apple. There is a big pulse at this point.

Effects: Cholera; vomiting; chest with full feeling and dyspena; swollen larynx; scrofula on neck.

Treatment: Needle: 1/8 to 1/4.
No deep needle it will kill the patient.
No Moxa.

Stimulus: Up to the jaw, down to the base of the neck.

Note: There is a big pulse here, be very careful to move pulse to the side before treating.

40.7 **Shui Tu** *water rushing* **ST-10**

Location: One division directly below ST-9.

Effects: Coughing; chi rushes up; pharynx swollen; dyspnea; cannot recline.

Treatment: Needle: 1/4 inch.
Moxa: 3 times.

Stimulus: Up to the ear and inwards to the throat.

40.8 **Chi She** *chi shelter* **ST-11**

Location: 1 division directly below ST-10; on the tip of the clavicle behind a tendon. One-half a division higher than CV-22.

Effects: Throat numb and swollen; neck stiff/painful; pharyngitis; throat swollen; goiter; skin tumor on the neck.

Treatment: Needle: 1/4 inch.
Moxa: 3 times.

Stimulus: Up to the temple and inwards to the throat.

40.9 **Chi Hu** *chi cottage* **ST-13**

Location: 4 divisions lateral to CV-21, between the clavicle and the first rib bone.

Effects: Coughing, chi rushes up the chest; pain on chest, which connects to the back with the coughing; loss of taste; anorexia; chest and ribs with a full sensation and dyspnea.

Treatment: Needle: 1/4 inch.
Moxa: 5 times.

Stimulus: Down to the side of the body close to the shoulder.

40.10 **Fu Fong** *treasure house* **ST-14**

Location: One intercostal space below ST-13, 4 divisions lateral to the Conception Vessel meridian (CV-20).

Effects: Full feelings in the chest/ribs; coughing and dyspnea; thick sputum with blood/pus.

Treatment: Needle: 1/4 inch.
Moxa: 5 times.

Stimulus: Down the chest and lateral to the arm.

40.11 **Wu Yi** *room screen* **ST-15**

Location: One intercostal space below ST-14; 4 divisions lateral to Conception Vessel meridian (CV-19), in the space between the 2nd and 3rd rib bones.

Effects: Coughing with chi rushing up; patient sorrowful; breast tumor.

Treatment: Needle: 1/4 inch or a little deeper.
Moxa: 5 times.

Stimulus: Down to the breast.

40.12 **Bu Yung** *no admittance* **ST-19**

Location: 2 divisions lateral to CV-14.

Effects: Full feeling in the upper abdomen; vomiting blood; shoulder/ribs painful; mouth dry; angina pectoris; pain on the shoulder radiating to the back; dyspnea; coughing; anorexia; borborygmi; vomiting with phlegm; gas moving in the abdomen.

Treatment: Needle: 1/4 inch or a little deeper.
Moxa: 5 times.

Stimulus: Local.

40.13 **Cheng Man** *receiving fullness* **ST-20**

Location: 2 divisions lateral to CV-13.

Effects: Borborygmi and full feelings in the abdomen; chi rushing up; anorexia; shoulders moving up and down during breathing; vomiting blood; sputum with thick phlegm/pus; whole body swollen; skin too painful to wear clothes; excessive secretion on the part of the female during intercourse.

Treatment: Needle: 1/4 inch or a little more.
Moxa: 5 times.

Stimulus: Local.

40.14 **Liang Men** *beam door* **ST-21**

Location: 2 divisions lateral to CV-12.

Effects: Gas under ribs at the sides of body; diarrhea with undigested food.

Treatment: Needle: 1/4 inch or a little more.
Moxa: 5 times.

Stimulus: Local.

40.15 **Guan Men** *gate door* **ST-22**

Location: 2 divisions lateral to CV-11.

Effects: Full feelings in the upper abdomen; borborygmi; intestinal pain; diarrhea; no appetite; gas running in the abdomen causing pain at the umbilicus; body swollen; chilled feelings; incontinence of urine.

Treatment: Needle: 1/2 inch.
Moxa: 5 times.

Stimulus: Local.

40.16 **Tai Yii** *bigger one* **ST-23**

Location: 2 divisions lateral to CV-10.

Effects: Patient walks about madly; melancholia; tongue stuck out.

Treatment: Needle: 1/2 inch.
Moxa: 5 times.

Stimulus: Local.

40.17 **Hua Rou Men** *slippery meat door* **ST-24**

Location: 2 divisions lateral to CV-9.

Effects: Madness; severe vomiting; tongue stiff; tongue stuck out.

Treatment: Needle: 1/2 inch.
Moxa: 5 times.

Stimulus: Local.

40.18 **Wai Ling** *outside hill* **ST-26**

Location: 2 divisions lateral to CV-7.

Effects: Pain in the upper abdomen; hanging sensation under the chest; pain radiating to the umbilicus.

Treatment: Needle: 1/2 inch.
Moxa: 5 times.

Stimulus: Felt approximately 3 divisions downward.

40.19 **Bi Guan** *thigh gate* **ST-31**

Location: 4 divisions lateral to LV-12 on top of the big muscle.

Effects: Lumbago; numbness of the thigh and knee with cold sensations; stiffness of upper thigh; cannot stretch; pain on lower abdomen radiating to the throat.

Treatment: Needle: 1/2 inch or a little more.
Moxa: 3 to 5 times.

Stimulus: Up to the top of the thigh and down approximately 5 inches.

40.20 **Fu Tu** *crouch rabbit* **ST-32**

Location: 6 divisions above the proximal border of the kneecap; also 3 divisions directly above ST-33, a little to the side of the center of the thigh.

Effects: Cold sensations in the knee; cramps on the arms; itching; eruptions; heavy sensations in the head; beri-beri.

Treatment: Needle: 1/2 inch.
No Moxa.

Stimulus: Down to the knee.

40.21 **Liang Chiu** *beam hill* **ST-34**

Location: 2 divisions above the kneecap at the outer corner of the thigh, one division below ST-33.

Effects: Pain on the knee and leg, lumbago with cold and numb sensations; patient kneels down and is unable to rise; both legs cold; breasts swollen and painful.

Treatment: Needle: 1/4 inch or a little more.
Moxa: 3 times.

Stimulus: Down to the kneecap.

40.22 **Du Bi** *calf nose* **ST-35**

Location: The outer "eye" of the knee, the outer hollow of the knee.

Effects: Pain on the knee; cannot bend or straighten; swollen knee; beri-beri.

Treatment: Needle: 1 inch.
Moxa: 5 times.

Stimulus: Up to the thigh and down the calf.

40.23 **Shang Ju Su** *upper great void* **ST-37**

Location: 3 divisions below ST-35; 1/4 division lateral to the tibia.

Effects: Beri-beri; numbness in back and leg; sore and painful tibia bone; difficult to bend, stretch, stand a long time; knee swollen; cold sensation in the bone marrow; indigestion in the large intestine caused by overcooling in the large intestine; diarrhea; pain in lower abdomen/loins; pain in the intestines; borborygmi; chi rushes up the chest; dyspnea; hot sensations in the stomach.

Treatment: Needle: 1/4 to 1/2 inch.
Moxa: 3 to 5 times.

Stimulus: Down to the foot.

40.24 **Tiao Kou** *line mouth* **ST-38**

Location: 2 divisions below ST-37; 1/4 division lateral to the tibia bone on the same level with ST-40.

Effects: Numbness in the leg; hot sensations in the leg, cannot stand; cold sensations in the leg and tibia; knee pain; leg pain; tibia area swollen; cramp of leg; drop foot.

Treatment: Needle: 1/4 to 1/2 inch.
Moxa: 3 to 5 times.

Stimulus: Reaction down to the foot.

40.25 **Sia Ju Su** *lower great void* **ST-39**

Location: One division below ST-38.

Effects: Pale face; weakness of legs; difficult to step on the floor; leg cold/numb; numbness in the throat; beri-beri; heavy feelings in the legs; dry lips; patient dribbling saliva; no perspiration; body hair dry/rough; after the flu, hot sensations in the stomach; no appetite; diarrhea with pus and blood; pain from chest to lower abdomen; hot sensations on the face in front of the ears; hot sensations in the shoulders or finger and small finger; madness and fearfulness with delirium and nonsensical speech; breast carbuncle (woman); drop foot; heel pain.

Treatment: Needle: 1/4 to 1/2 inch.
Moxa: 3 to 5 times.

Stimulus: Down to the foot.

40.26 **Shian Gu** *sinking valley* **ST-43**

Location: Between the second and third metatarsal bones; 1/2 division behind the joint.

Effects: Dropsy with swollen face; belching; borborygmi; gastric pain; high fever with chills and no perspiration.

Treatment: Needle: 1/4 inch.
Moxa: 3 times.

Stimulus: Down to the second toe.

Section 41 **Gall Bladder Meridian**

41.1 **Shang Guan** *upper gate* **GB-3**

Location: 1 and 1/2 eye divisions in front of TW-21, on the upper edge of the cheek bone, directly above ST-7.

Effects: Stiffness of the upper lip; one side of the face paralyzed; cataract in eye; dim vision; fear of the cold wind; tooth decay; jaw cramp, unable to chew; tinnitus; deafness.

Treatment: **No Needle.**
Moxa: 3 times.
Deep needle here would cause deafness.

Stimulus: Up to the temple.

41.2 **Han Yan** *jaw detested* **GB-4**

Location: 2 divisions above XF-3 Yin Tang, lateral one division past hairline in the horizontal and vertical cleft.

Effects: Migraine headache; pain on one side of head and neck; pain in the eyes; convulsions in children; tinnitus; dimness of eyes; pain and tightness in the outer canthus; excessive sneezing; pain in the arm joints; both arms and hands tired.

Treatment: Needle: 1/8 to 1/4 inch.
Moxa: 3 times.
No deep needle; deep needle might cause deafness.

Stimulus: Around the temple to the forehead.

41.3 **Shuan Lu** *suspended skull* **GB-5**

Location: One division above XF-3, Yin Tang, between eyebrows; lateral one division past the hairline in the horizontal and vertical cleft.

Effects: Headache; face swollen; fever without perspiration; migraine headache causing the outer canthus to be red/painful; thick mucus from the nose.

Treatment: Needle: 1/8 to 1/4 inch.
Moxa: 3 times.
No deep needle, deep needle would cause deafness.

Stimulus: Around the temple area.

41.4 **Shuan Li** *suspended balance* **GB-6**

Location: Directly lateral to the end of the eyebrow; one division past the hairline at the horizontal/vertical cleft.

Effects: Face red and swollen; migraine headaches; melancholia and anorexia; high fever without perspiration; red/painful outer canthus.

Treatment: Needle: 1/4 inch.
Moxa: 3 times.

Stimulus: Up to the temple and the side of the head.

41.5 **Chu Bin** *twisted hair* **GB-7**

Location: Lateral to a point midway between the outer canthus and the end of the eyebrow, one division past the hairline in the horizontal cleft.

Effects: Upper jaw swollen, preventing the mouth from opening, the patient from talking; stiffness of the neck, cannot turn; headache on one side of the head; face paralyzed, causing dimness of the eyes.

Treatment: Needle: 1/4 inch.
Moxa: 3 to 7 times.

Stimulus: Up to one side of the head and forward to the temple.

41.6 **Shuai Gu** *leading valley* **GB-8**

Location: One half the length of the patient's ear directly above the apex of the helix, at the horizontal/vertical cleft.

Effects: Headache on one side; pain on the top of the head; vomiting; melancholia; drunkenness; skin swollen; overcooling with phlegm in the stomach.

Treatment: Needle: 1/4 inch.
Moxa: 3 times.

Stimulus: Into the head and down to the temple.

41.7 **Tien Chung** *heavenly rushing* **GB-9**

Location: One half division behind GB-8 in the vertical cleft.

Effects: Insanity; gums swollen; patient frightened.

Treatment: Needle: 1/4 inch.
Moxa: 3 times.

Stimulus: Down to the ear up the side of the head.

41.8 **Fu Bai** *floating white* **GB-10**

Location: In a vertical cleft directly below GB-9 and approximately 3/4 of an eye division from the helix.

Effects: Difficulty walking because of the legs; deafness; tinnitus; toothache; chest with full feeling/difficult breathing; chest painful; scrofula or neck tumor preventing speech; difficulty raising the arm/shoulder; tonsillitis; coughing with phlegm; tinnitus causing deafness.

Treatment: Needle: 1/4 inch.
Moxa: 3 to 7 times.

Stimulus: : Up the side of the head and down the back of the ear.

41.9 **Chiao Yin** *the yin of a hole* **GB-11**

Location: Up two-thirds the length of the ear, behind the edge of the helix 2/3 of an eye division, in the horizontal cleft.

Effects: Four limbs cramped; eye pain; pain on one side of the head, neck/jaw; tinnitus causing deafness; bleeding on the tongue; carbuncle on the bone; hot sensations on hands and feet without perspiration; stiffness of the neck; coughing; intercostal neuralgia; throat inflamed; bitter taste in the mouth.

Treatment: Needle: 1/8 to 1/4 inch.
Moxa: 3 to 7 times.

Stimulus: Up to the temple and the back of the head.

41.10 **Wan Ku** *final bone* **GB-12**

Location: Almost one division lateral to GB-20; at the base of the skull between 2 muscles.

Effects: Drop foot; jaw cramped and swollen; head and face swollen; neck pain; pain behind the ear; melancholia; icteric or red urine; toothache; facial paralysis; insanity; headaches.

Treatment: Needle: 1/4 inch or a little more.
Moxa: 3 times.

Stimulus: Down to neck and up to the temple.

41.11 **Cheng Ying** *upright camp* **GB-17**

Location: 1 and 1/2 divisions behind GB-16.

Effects: Dizziness and dimness of the eye; migraine headache associated with the neck; toothache; lips stiff.

Treatment: Needle: 1/4 inch.
Moxa: 5 times.

Stimulus: Up one side of the head.

41.12 **Cheng Ling** *receiving spirit* **GB-18**

Location: 1 and 1/2 divisions behind GB-17.

Effects: Headache on top of the head; patient afraid of the cold wind; nose stuffed/bleeding; dyspnea.

Treatment: **No Needle.**
Moxa: 3 times.

Stimulus: Around the local area.

41.13 **Nao Kong** *brain hollow* **GB-19**

Location: 1 and 1/2 divisions above GB-20 in the horizontal/vertical cleft.

Effects: Tuberculosis; body emaciated and feverish; neck stiff, cannot turn; severe headache with heavy feelings on one side of the head; eyelids with heavy feelings; heart palpitations; nose pain.

Treatment: Needle: 1/4 inch.
Moxa: 3 times.

Stimulus: Around one side of the back of the head.

41.14 **Yuan Yeh** *liquid of deep waters* **GB-22**

Location: 4 divisions lateral to ST-16, under the armpit between two ribs.

Effects: Carbuncle under the armpit; full feelings in the chest with weakness; cannot raise the arm.

Treatment: Needle: 1/4 inch.
No Moxa.

Stimulus: Down the side of the chest.

Note: Moxa will cause a carbuncle to grow. If the carbuncle breaks on the inside, the patient will die.

41.15 **Che Jin** *flank muscle* **GB-23**

Location: Between the same rib bones as GB-22, in front of GB-22 1 and 1/4 divisions.

Effects: Chest suddenly feels full; patient cannot sleep or breathe; patient crying and easily worried; hot sensation in the lower abdomen; excessive spitting; speech difficult; four limbs weak; vomiting.

Treatment: Needle: 1/4 to 1/2 inch.
Moxa: 3 times.

Stimulus: Reaction up the armpit.

41.16 **Yih Yueh** *sun and moon* **GB-24**

Location: One intercostal space directly below LV-14.

Effects: Sighing; patient cries easily; hot sensations in the lower abdomen; excessive spitting; speech difficult; four limbs weak.

Treatment: Needle: 1/4 to 1/2 inch.
Moxa: 5 times.

Stimulus: Up the chest.

41.17 **Jing Men** *capital door* **GB-25**

Location: Behind the tip of the 12th rib, on the back.

Effects: Borborygmi; lower abdomen painful; cramps and cold sensations in the shoulders and back; numbness/pain on the shoulder; lumbar ache; patient cannot bend or stand; cold and hot body sensations, causing the abdomen to swell, the back to ache and dyspnea; dysuria; icteric urine; lower abdomen cramp; diarrhea; pain on the hip radiating to the lower abdomen.

Treatment: Needle: 1/4 to 1/2 inch.
Moxa: 3 to 5 times.

Stimulus: Felt in the lower abdomen.

41.18 **Wu Shu** *five pivots* **GB-27**

Location: 6 divisions lateral to CV-4.

Effects: Loins and back painful; testicles retracted into the body; red and white vaginal discharge; false call to stool.

Treatment: Needle: 1/2 to 3/4 inch .
Moxa: 5 times.

Stimulus: Down to the lower abdomen.

41.19 **Wei Dao** *blinding path* **GB-28**

Location: 5 and 1/2 divisions lateral from between CV-4 and CV-3 and 1/2 division below GB-27.

Effects: Vomiting; ceaseless vomiting; edema; anorexia.

Treatment: Needle: 1/2 to 3/4 inch.
Moxa: 3 times.

Stimulus: Down to the lower abdomen.

41.20 **Ju Liao** *dwelling bone* **GB-29**

Location: With the leg bent at a 90 degree angle the point is on the iliac side of the greater trochanter of the femur opposite GB-30.

Effects: Back pain radiating to the lower abdomen; shoulder pain radiating to the chest immobilizing the arm.

Treatment: Needle: 3/4 to 1 inch.
Moxa: 3 times.

Stimulus: Down to the middle of the thigh.

41.21 **Jung Du** *middle ditch* **GB-32**

Location: 5 divisions directly above GB-33 (from the posterior knee crease on the middle of the thigh).

Effects: Sciatica; loins and legs painful; general weakness of the leg; legs numb.

Treatment: Needle: 1/2 inch or a little deeper.
Moxa: 5 times.

Stimulus: Down to the knee.

41.22 **Yang Jiao** *yang crossing* **GB-35**

Location: 7 divisions directly above the upper edge of the lateral malleolus in front of the fibula.

Effects: Chest full and swollen; knee pain; drop foot; throat numb; face swollen; cold feet.

Treatment: Needle: A little more than 1 inch.
Moxa: 3 to 5 times.

Stimulus: Down to the foot.

41.23 **Wai Chiu** *outer mound* **GB-36**

Location: One finger division directly behind GB-35 on the fibula.

Effects: Full feelings on the chest; skin painful; neck painful; patient dislikes wind and cold; insanity; hunchback with the sternum also protruding; for rabies, three different people from different families must burn moxa on this point.

Treatment: Needle: 1/4 to 1/2 inch.
Moxa: 3 times.

Stimulus: Down to the ankle.

41.24 **Guang Ming** *light bright* **GB-37**

Location: 5 divisions above the upper edge of the lateral malleolus in front of the fibula.

Effects: Female secretes excessive liquid during/before intercourse; fibula painful; patient cannot stand for a long period of time; high fever without perspiration; acute insanity; drop foot; knee painful; baby clenches teech; all eye diseases.

Treatment: Needle: 1/2 to 3/4 inch.
Moxa: 5 times.

Stimulus: Down to the toes.

41.25 **Lin Chi** *(foot) above tears* **GB-41**

Location: One division proximal to the joint, between the 4th and 5th metatarsal bones.

Effects: Full feeling in the chest; carbuncles behind the clavicle and in the armpit; excessive secretions on the part of the female during intercourse; tibia sore; eyes dizzy; pain on the base of the skull; pain in the chest with chills; leg painful in different areas at different times; dyspnea and difficulty walking; malaria; irregular menses; rib bone area swollen; breast with carbuncle.

Treatment: Needle: 1/4 inch.
Moxa: 3 times.

Stimulus: Down to the toes.

41.26 **Di Wu Hui** *earth five meetings* **GB-42**

Location: 1/2 division proximal to the joint between the 4th and 5th metatarsals.

Effects: Pain under the armpit; coughing with blood; dry skin on the legs; breast carbuncle.

Treatment: Needle: 1/4 inch.
No Moxa.

Stimulus: Down to the toes.

41.27 **Shia Shi** *chivalrous stream* **GB-43**

Location: Between the 4th and 5th metatarsals between the joint and the web.

Effects: Chest pain; the flu with a high fever and no perspiration; outer canthus red; jaw swollen; deafness; chest pain, the patient cannot turn the body; pain on chest in different areas at different times.

Treatment: Needle: 1/4 inch.
Moxa: 3 times.

Stimulus: Down to the toes.

Section 42 **Bladder Meridian**

42.1 **Mei Chung** *eyebrow raising* **BL-3**

Location: Directly above BL-2 past the hairline one-half division; also one-half division lateral to GV-24.

Effects: Headaches; eyes dizzy; nose stuffed; anosmia; epilepsy.

Treatment: Needle: 1/8 inch.
Moxa: 3 times.

Stimulus: Down to the forehead.

42.2 **Chu Cha** *crooked officer* **BL-4**

Location: Traditionally 1 division lateral to GV-24 in the third cleft from the center line.

Effects: Eye dimness; epistaxis; stuffed nose; nasal abscess; melancholia; headache on the top of the head; top of the head swollen; fever without perspiration.

Treatment: Needle: 1/8 inch.
Moxa: 3 times.

Stimulus: Reaction down the forehead.

42.3 **Wu Chu** *five places* **BL-5**

Location: 1 division lateral to GV-23 in the second cleft from the center line.

Effects: Cramping on the spine; head tilted up; insanity with total body cramping; hot sensations in the head; eye dizziness; dim vision; eyes locked looking upwards.

Treatment: Needle: 1/8 inch.
Moxa: 3 times.

Stimulus: To the forehead.

42.4 **Cheng Kuang** *receive light* **BL-6**

Location: 1 and 1/2 divisions directly behind BL-5.

Effects: Dizziness; headache; vomiting; melancholia; stuffed nose; anosmia; facial paralysis; runny nose; film over the eyes.

Treatment: Needle: 1/8 inch.
No Moxa.

Stimulus: To the forehead.

42.5 **Tung Tien** *penetrate heaven* **BL-7**

Location: 1 and 1/2 divisions behind BL-6, which is also lateral to a point one division in front of GV-20, in the third cleft.

Effects: Stiffness of the neck; epistaxis; stuffed nose; vertigo; shock; facial paralysis; dyspnea; heavy feeling in the head; goiter.

Treatment: Needle: 1/8 inch.
Moxa: 3 times.

Stimulus: Down to the forehead.

42.6 **Lo Chueh** *connecting deficient* **BL-8**

Location: 1 and 1/2 divisions behind BL-7, which is also lateral to a point 1/2 division behind GV-20, in the third cleft.

Effects: Dizziness; tinnitus; patient runs around madly; cramps; patient unhappy and distant from reality; abdomen swollen.

Treatment: Needle: 1/8 inch.
Moxa: 3 times.

Stimulus: Down the back of the head.

42.7 **Yu Jeen** *jade pillow* **BL-9**

Location: Lateral 1 and 1/2 divisions to GV-17 in the third cleft; also two divisions above the back hairline.

Effects: Severe eye pain; myopia; severe headache; stuffed nose and anosmia.

Treatment: Needle: 1/4 inch
Moxa: 3 times.

Stimulus: Up the back of the head and down to the hairline.

42.8 **Chuh Yin Yu** *absolute yin yu* **BL-14**

Location: Lateral 1 and 1/2 divisions to the 4th intervertebral space.

Effects: Coughing; toothache; angina pectoris; full feeling in the chest; vomiting; melancholia; point for the pericardium (pericardium yu).

Treatment: Needle: 1/4 to 1/2 inch.
Moxa: 7 times.

Stimulus: To the sides of the body.

42.9 **Du Yu** *governing vessel yu* **BL-16**

Location: Lateral 1 and 1/2 divisions to the 6th intervertebral space.

Effects: Cardiac pain; dilatation of the heart; abdomen pain; borborygmi; chi rushes up the abdomen to the chest; fever with shivering.

Treatment: Needle: 1/4 to 1/2 inch.
Moxa: 3 to 5 times.

Stimulus: To the side of the body.

42.10 **Chi Hai Yu** *sea of chi yu* **BL-24**

Location: Lateral 1 and 1/2 divisions to the intervertebral space between the third and fourth lumbar vertebrae.

Effects: Lumbago; hemorrhoids; anal fistula.

Treatment: Needle: 1/2 to 3/4 inch.
Moxa: 5 times.

Stimulus: Slanting down to the outside of the buttocks.

42.11 **Guan Yuan Yu** *gate origin yu* **BL-26**

Location: Lateral 1 and 1/2 divisions to the space between the fifth lumbar vertebrae and the sacrum.

Effects: Lumbago; diarrhea; inflammation of the rectum; dysuria; gas, like a stone in the abdomen, but moving (when found in a woman).

Treatment: Needle: 1/2 to 3/4 inch.
Moxa: 3 to 5 times.

Stimulus: Down to the buttocks.

42.12 **Jung Lu Yu**

middle of the backbone yu **BL-29**

Location: Lateral 1 and 1/2 divisions to the intervertebral space between the third and fourth sacral vertebrae.

Effects: Lumbago; pain on the sides of the vertebra from the neck to the sacrum; kidneys weak; spine stiff; cannot bend or rise; thirst; intestines with cold sensations; red or white dysentery; abdominal pain; abdomen swollen; loin pain.

Treatment: Needle: 1/2 inch or a little more.
Moxa: 3 to 5 times.

Stimulus: Down to the bottom of the buttocks.

42.13 **Fu Fen** *supplementary division* **BL-36**

Location: Three divisions lateral to the number 2 intervertebral space; 1 and 1/2 divisions lateral to BL-12.

Effects: Shoulder and elbow numb; shoulder cramp radiating to the back; cold on the back; neck pain (cannot turn).

Treatment: Needle: 1/4 inch or a little more.
Moxa: 5 times.

Stimulus: Up to the shoulder and neck.

42.14 **Po Hu** *strength house* **BL-37**

Location: 3 divisions lateral to GV-12; 1 and 1/2 divisions lateral to BL-13.

Effects: Pain on the shoulder; lungs withered (overcooled); neck stiff; cannot turn the head; coughing; vomiting; melancholia.

Treatment: Needle: 1/4 to 1/2 inch.
Moxa: 7 to 100 times.

Stimulus: Up to the shoulder and neck.

42.15 **Shen Tang** *spirit hall* **BL-39**

Location: 3 divisions lateral to GV-11.

Effects: Back stiff; patient cannot bend backwards or forwards; chills and fevers; full feelings in the chest with the chi rushing up, belching.

Treatment: Needle: 1/4 to 1/2 inch.
Moxa: 5 times.

Stimulus: Up to the shoulder, down to the sides of the back.

42.16 **Yi Shi** *sighing giggling* **BL-40**

Location: 3 divisions lateral to GV-10.

Effects: Fever without perspiration; weakness of the body with insomnia; malaria; melancholia (chest); full feeling in abdomen; pain in the chest reacting to the back; pain in the ribs; eyes painful and dizzy; epistaxis; dyspnea; pain on shoulder/arm; child gets a headache from eating.

Treatment: Needle: 1/4 to 1/2 inch.
Moxa: 5 times.

Stimulus: Down to the loins.

42.17 **Ge Guan** *diaphragm gate* **BL-41**

Location: 3 divisions lateral to GV-9.

Effects: Pain on the back with chills; stiffness of the back; difficult to bend forwards and backwards; patient cannot eat or drink; vomiting; excessive spitting; melancholia; frequent bowel movements; urine icteric.

Treatment: Needle: 1/4 inch or a little more.
Moxa: 5 times.

Stimulus: Down to the sides of the back.

42.18 **Hwen Men** *soul door* **BL-42**

Location: 3 divisions lateral to GV-8.

Effects: Shock; pain in chest radiating to the back; food and drink do not decend; borborygmi; frequency of bowel movement; urine icteric.

Treatment: Needle: 1/4 inch or a little more.
Moxa: 3 times.

Stimulus: To the sides of the back.

42.19 **Yang Gang** *yang bound* **BL-43**

Location: 3 divisions lateral to GV-7.

Effects: Borborygmi; gastric pain; food and drink do not decend; dysuria and hematuria; abdomen swollen with fever; excessive bowel movements; yellow/red dysentery; anorexia; body lazy.

Treatment: Needle 1/4 inch or a little more.
Moxa: 3 to 7 times.

Stimulus: To the sides of the body.

42.20 **Yi Sheh** *thought shelter* **BL-44**

Location: 3 divisions lateral to GV-6.

Effects: Abdomen swollen with gas; diarrhea; urine icteric, red; back pain; patient hates the wind and the cold; vomiting; thirst; jaundice and fever.

Treatment: Needle: 1/4 to 1/2 inch.
Moxa: 5 to 50 times.

Stimulus: To the sides of the body.

42.21 **Wei Tsang** *stomach granary* **BL-45**

Location: 1 and 1/2 divisions lateral to BL-21.

Effects: Abdomen swollen with gas; patient cannot eat or drink; chills; pain on the back; cannot bend backwards or forwards.

Treatment: Needle: 1/4 to 1/2 inch.
Moxa: 5 times.

Stimulus: Felt down to one side of the body.

42.22 **Huang Men** *vitals door* **BL-46**

Location: 3 divisions lateral to GV-5 between the first and second lumbar vertebrae.

Effects: Severe pain under the chest; feces too dry; breast disease in women.

Treatment: Needle: 1/4 to 1/2 inch.
Moxa: 5 to 30 times.

Stimulus: Down to the buttocks.

42.23 **Bao Huang** *womb and vitals* **BL-48**

Location: 3 divisions lateral to the intervertebral space under the second sacral vertebrae; 1 and 1/2 divisions lateral to BL-28.

Effects: Acute pain in the lumbar area; indigestion; hardness in the abdomen; borborygmi; retention of urine.

Treatment: Needle: 1/2 inch.
Moxa: 3 to 21 times.

Stimulus: Down to the hip.

42.24 **Jih Bian** *folding edge* **BL-49**

Location: 3 divisions lateral to the intervertebral space below the fourth sacral vertebra, 1 and 1/2 divisions lateral to BL-30.

Effects: Lumbago; chronic hemorrhoids; swelling/pain on the buttocks; constipation; dysuria.

Treatment: Needle: 1 inch or a little more.
Moxa: 5 times.

Stimulus: Down to the back of the thigh.

42.25 **Yi Men** *prosperous gate* **BL-51**

Location: 6 divisions directly below BL-50, in the center of the back of the thigh.

Effects: Pain in back and loins; cannot bend the back, or stand straight up; hemorrhage of the rectum; thighs swollen.

Treatment: Needle: 1/2 to 3/4 inch.
No Moxa.

Stimulus: Down towards the foot.

42.26 **Fu Shi** *floating accumulation* **BL-52**

Location: One division above BL-53.

Effects: Cramping from cholera; overheating in the small intestines; hot sensations from urination; dry feces in the intestines; cramps in the calf; numbness in the hip joint.

Treatment: Needle: 1/2 inch.
Moxa: 3 times.

Stimulus: Down to the calf.

42.27 **Wei Yang** *commanding yang* **BL-53**

Location: On the back knee crease, towards the outside of the leg, between the big and small tendon.

Effects: Pain/swelling under the armpit; chest with full feelings; muscular spasms in general; fever; numbness in the legs; urinary incontinence.

Treatment: Needle: 1/2 inch.
Moxa: 3 times.

Stimulus: Down to the foot.

42.28 **Ho Yang** *uniting yang* **BL-55**

Location: 2 divisions directly below BL-54, in between 2 muscles.

Effects: Hernia; stiffness on back and spine with pain radiating to the abdomen; hot sensations in the inner thigh; tibia bone area swollen and sore; walking difficult; pain on one side of the vagina; menorrhagia.

Treatment: Needle: 1/2 inch.
Moxa: 5 times.

Stimulus: Down to the foot.

42.29 **Cheng Jin** *supporting nerves* **BL-56**

Location: 5 divisions directly below BL-54 in between two muscles.

Effects: Stiffness of the back; constipation; swelling under the armpit; hemorrhoids; thigh and leg numb; thigh sore; leg stiff; heel pain; lumbago; epistaxis; cholera with cramping.

Treatment: **No Needle.**
Moxa: 3 to 5 times.

Stimulus: Down to the heel.

42.30 **Fei Yang** *flying high* **BL-58**

Location: One division below BL-57, one-half a division lateral to the outside of the calf between two muscles.

Effects: Hemorrhoids painful/swollen; whole body feels heavy; difficulty sitting down, standing up; calf pain; person shakes while standing and cannot stand for a long time; after sitting a long time the toes cannot move; dizziness/pain in the eyes; general joint pain; madness; headaches and epistaxis associated with malaria.

Treatment: Needle: 1/4 to 1/2 inch.
Moxa: 3 to 5 times.

Stimulus: Down to the foot.

42.31 **Fu Yang** *foot bone yang* **BL-59**

Location: 3 divisions directly above BL-60.

Effects: Cramping associated with cholera; lumbago; difficulty standing for a long time or difficulty standing up after sitting; hip and thigh pain; leg numb and becoming withered; head heavy and painful; fevers and chills; canot raise the four limbs.

Treatment: Needle: 1/2 inch.
Moxa: 3 to 5 times.

Stimulus: Down to the small toes.

42.32 **Pu Tsan** *official's aide* **BL-61**

Location: 2 divisions below BL-60, 1/4 of a division towards the back of the heel in the cleft on the heel bone.

Effects: Drop foot; heel pain; cramping associated with cholera; vomiting; shock; insanity with hallucinations; beri-beri; knee swollen.

Treatment: Needle: 1/8 inch.
Moxa: 3 to 7 times.

Stimulus: Around the heel area.

42.33 **Jing Gu** *capital bone* **BL-64**

Location: 2 divisions proximal to the head of the 5th metatarsal bone on the outer side of the foot where the yin and yang skin meet.

Effects: Severe headaches; lumbago; patient cannot bend; inner canthus red/painful; white spot over the iris; eyes dizzy; malaria; patient frightened; anorexia; epistaxis; leg cramps; leg pain; neck stiffness; loosening energy on the spine; cardiac pain.

Treatment: Needle: 1/4 inch or a little more.
Moxa: 3 to 5 times.

Stimulus: Down to the small toes.

42.34 **Shu Gu** *bind the bone* **BL-65**

Location: Just proximal to the head of the fifth metatarsal bone, behind the joint, on the side of the foot where the yin and yang skin meet.

Effects: Severe back pain; cannot bend the hips; stiffness behind the knee; deafness; hatred of the wind; headache radiating to the jaw and neck; eye dizziness; eyes jaundiced; excess tearing; muscles twitching; neck stiff; cannot turn head; inner canthus red/painful; diarrhea; hemorrhoids; madness; poisonous furuncle on the back.

Treatment: Needle: 1/4 inch.
Moxa: 3 times.

Stimulus: Locally and to the small toes.

42.35 **Tung Gu** *penetrating the valley* **BL-66**

Location: Just distal to the head of the 5th metatarsal in front of the joint, on the side of the foot, on top of the bone.

Effects: Heavy feeling in the head; eye dizziness; paranoia; epistaxis; neck stiffness; dim vision; water stagnates in the stomach; indigestion.

Treatment: Needle: 1/8 inch.
Moxa: 3 times.

Stimulus: Locally.

Index

There are four indexes in this section. The first index lists points contraindicated for needle and moxa. The second index is the general index which references effects or indications for the use of all of the points discussed in the text. This index is organized such that a search for a particular reference should begin with a general category such as "swelling," then proceed to a specific body area. For example, "swelling of the abdomen" will be found in the index section "swelling." To avoid repeated searches, subjects are listed in context; for example, "cough," "cough with pain in the chest" and "cough with fever." Disease names (e.g. cholera), symptoms (e.g. dry tongue) and Chinese energetic concepts (e.g. overheating), are intermixed alphabetically. The section on pain is divided into body areas and items are listed specifically within each area.

Once you are familiar with each of the points, the general index may be used as a reference without returning to the text. Each index entry includes both the point number and the page number. Thus, "CV-23, 11; GB-15, 14" indicates that CV-23 and GB-15 have been noted in regard to the indexed effect, and are discussed on pages 11 and 14 respectively. Points indexed to the same indication are not necessarily points which should be used in combination, please refer to Dr. So's **Treatment of Disease by Acupuncture** for combinations and treatments.

The third index cross references all of the notations in regard to pain. This is a "permuted index" which differs from the usual indexing style. Selected key words such as ache, pain, lumbago, neuralgia and sciatica are found in the center column of the page. The specific context in which these key words were used in the text appears to the right of the key with any additional context appearing in the left margin. This index may be used for quick, yet specific searches of the many effects listed in the text which refer to pain.

The final index lists each of the points discussed. Two identifications are listed for all points, and a third is included for most. The first numbers shown are the section and sub-section number for the point. The second is the number of the illustration where the point is shown and the last is the page number of the point discussion. The illustration number is absent if no specific illustration of the point has been included. The points are organized by meridian.

Contraindications

Point	Contraindication	Illus.	Page
BL-1	Moxa	8	26
BL-2	Moxa	8	25
BL-6	Needle		237
BL-49	Needle		246
BL-51	Moxa		244
BL-54	Moxa		155
BL-56	Needle		246
BL-60	Needle, during pregnancy	29	158
BL-62	Moxa	29	158
BL-67	Needle, during pregnancy	29	159
CV-4	Moxa, during pregnancy	15	60
CV-4	Moxa, wet dreams	15	60
CV-4	Needle, during pregnancy	15	60
CV-5	Moxa, women	15	59
CV-5	Needle, women	15	59
CV-8	Needle	14	55
CV-11	Moxa, during pregnancy	14	53
CV-14	Deep needle	14	52
CV-15	Needle	14	51
CV-17	Needle	12	43
GB-1	Moxa	8	27
GB-3	Deep needle		224
GB-4	Deep needle		224
GB-5	Deep needle		225
GB-15	Moxa, will cause blindness	5	14
GB-18	Needle		228
GB-21	Deep needle, heart problems	17	71
GB-21	Needle, pregnancy	17	71
GB-21	Needle, with heart problems	17	71
GB-22	Moxa		229
GB-33	Moxa	30	162
GB-42	Moxa		235
GV-4	Moxa, in young males	18	78
GV-6	Moxa		171
GV-11	Needle	18	76
GV-15	Deep needle	6	18
GV-15	Moxa	6	18
GV-16	Moxa, loss of speech	6	17
GV-17	Needle, Moxa	30	172

GV-23	Moxa (more than 5)	5	11
GV-24	Needle, at evening	5	11
GV-24	Needle, may cause madness	5	11
GV-25	Moxa	9	29
GV-26	Moxa, will cause death	10	31
GV-28	Moxa	30	173
HT-2	Needle		177
KI-11	Needle		197
LI-15	Moxa, limited use only	17	72
LI-19	Moxa		184
LI-20	Moxa	9	29
LI-4	Needle, during pregnancy	22	115
LU-2	Needle		174
LU-3	Moxa		174
LU-5	Moxa	21	99
LU-8	Moxa	21	101
LU-10	Moxa		176
LU-11	Moxa	21	102
LU-52	Needle, more than twice	21	106
LU-52	Needle, with nasal polyps	21	106
LV-12	Needle		212
PC-9	Moxa	21	107
SI-10	Moxa	24	129
SI-11	Needle	24	130
SI-18	Moxa		195
SP-2	Moxa, pregnancy and after	25	132
SP-6	Needle, pregnant woman	25	134
SP-7	Moxa		204
ST-1	Needle		213
ST-2	Deep needle		213
ST-2	Needle		213
ST-7	Moxa		215
ST-8	Moxa, may cause blindness	6	16
ST-9	Deep needle		215
ST-17	Needle, Moxa		
ST-25	Needle, during pregnancy	16	66
ST-32	Moxa		220
TW-7	Needle		185
TW-8	Needle		185
TW-16	Needle		188
TW-19	Bleeding Forbidden		189

TW-23	Moxa	8	26
XA-2	Needle	24	127
XB-1	Needle	20	96
XF-4	Moxa	11	38
XF-5	Moxa	11	38
XF-6	Moxa	11	38
XF-7	Moxa	11	38
XF-8	Moxa	11	38
XFi-2	Needle	24	128
XFi-3	Needle	24	128
XFi-4	Moxa	24	129
XH-1	Needle	11	34
XL-2	Needle	28	149
XL-3	Needle	29	157
XN-10	Moxa	11	38
XN-11	Moxa	11	38
XN-12	Moxa	11	39
XN-14	Moxa	11	39
XP-1	Moxa	15	64
XSC-1	Needle	15	63
XT-1	Needle		153

General Index

Abdomen

See also: swelling, pain
abdomen and the sides of the body painful, SP-8, 205
abdomen distended, BL-23, 88; CV-10, 54; GV-6, 171; KI-16, 199; SP-12, 206; CV-10, 54; CV-12, 53; CV-4, 60; CV-6, 58
abdomen distended and borborygmus, BL-22, 87
abdomen, hard mass (dish), CV-13, 52
abdomen, hardness in, BL-48, 244
abdomen painful, BL-16, 239; BL-29, 240; CV-10, 54; KI-17, 199; KI-5, 196; SP-13, 206; CV-11, 53
abdomen painful after confinement, CV-4, 60
abdomen painful down to the sexual organs, CV-4, 60
abdomen swollen, BL-21, 86; BL-29, 240; BL-8, 238; ST-41, 151; ST-42, 152
abdomen swollen and breathing difficult, KI-10, 197
abdomen swollen like a drum, CV-12, 53; CV-10, 54; CV-4, 60; CV-6,58
abdomen swollen, painful, hot, CV-5, 59
abdomen swollen (fever), BL-43, 242
abdomen swollen with gas, BL-44, 243; BL-45, 243; ST-36, 150
abdomen swollen, with panting, CV-6, 58
abdomen swollen with worms, gas or tumor (female), KI-1, 141
abdominal cramps, BL-47, 97
abdominal tumor, SP-6, 134

Abscess

abscess, SP-10, 135
abscess in the ear, TW-21, 21
abscess in the larynx, CV-22, 42
abscess in the mouth, CV-23, 41; 39
abscess in area of sexual organs, BL-28, 90; BL-47, 97
abscess in the finger web, TW-6, 123
abscess of the nose, ST-3, 214
abundant stools, KI-14, 198
acne, LI-11, 118; LU-2, 174
adenitis, PC-1, 178
allergic rhinorrhea, BL-2, 25

Amenorrhea

amenorrhea, BL-23, 88; CV-4, 60; GV-2, 79; KI-7, 145; LV-3, 138; ST-28, 67; ST-29, 68
amenorrhea in young women, CV-1, 62
anal fistula, BL-24, 239; SI-16, 194
anal hemmorrhaging, BL-57, 157
anal prolapse, BL-35, 93
anemia of the brain, GV-20, 13; GV-21, 12
anemic after confinement, SP-6, 134
anemic headache, GV-22, 12
angry and scolding patient, ST-36, 150
anger and excessive talking, KI-8, 146

Angina

See also: cardiac, heart
angina pectoris, CV-6, 58; ST-36, 150; TW-6, 123; BL-14, 238; CV-15, 51; HT-4, 109; HT-6, 110; HT-7, 111; HT-9, 113; KI-1, 141; LV-3, 138; PC-3, 103; PC-4, 103; PC-6, 105; PC-7, 105; PC-9, 107; ST-19, 217; XT-1, 153
angina pectoris (acute), CV-6, 58; ST-36, 150; KI-3, 143; TW-6, 123
ankle joint painful, KI-6, 144
ankle pain (severe), BL-60, 158
anorexia, BL-17, 84; BL-20, 86; BL-22, 87; BL-43, 242; BL-64, 248; CV-10, 54; CV-11, 53; CV-12, 53; GB-28, 232; GB-6, 225; GV-6, 171; KI-17, 199; KI-21, 201; KI-22, 201; KI-23, 201; KI-24, 202; KI-25, 202; KI-26, 202; KI-27, 203; SP-8, 205; SP-9, 135; ST-13, 216; ST-19, 217; ST-20, 218; TW-10, 186; GB-39, 164; ST-42, 152
anorexia in children, HT-8, 112; XFi-1, 113
anorexic malaria, ST-45, 153
anosmia, BL-3, 236; BL-6, 237; KI-24, 202; LI-19, 184; LI-20, 29
anuria, BL-30, 90; BL-31, 91; BL-32, 91; BL-34, 92; BL-54, 155; KI-11, 197; LV-8, 139; SP-11, 205; SP-6, 134; ST-36, 150
anuria with swelling of the bladder, CV-8, 55
aphasia, 14, 39
aphonia, CV-22, 42

Apoplexy

See also: stroke.
apoplexy with perspiration, LU-5, 99
apoplexy, GB-15, 14; GV-15, 18; GV-26, 31
apoplexy patient cannot talk with paralysis of tongue, GV-16, 17
appendix, point especially powerful for inflammation of, ST-36a, 150
appetite, See also: emaciation, anorexia
appetite poor, GV-20, 13; ST-22, 218; ST-39, 222; CV-9, 54; SP-4, 133; SP-6, 134; ST-36, 150

Arm

See also: pain, swelling, inflammation
arm and elbow, weakness of, TW-5, 123
arm and hand tired, HT-8, 112
cannot raise arm, GB-21, 71; GB-22, 229; KI-22, 201; LI-15, 72; LU-2, 174; LV-13, 48; SI-12, 193; SI-14, 186; TW-2, 121; SI-10, 192; TW-14, 187; HT-2, 177
arm, cannot raise shoulder and arm, LI-16, 72
arm, cramped difficult to stretch, SI-7, 192
arm, cramping or numb, LI-12, 182
arm, difficulty in raising the arm, LU-5, 99
arm pain, LI-12, 182; LI-14, 119; SI-2, 191; TW-13, 187 LU-6, 175
arm, weakness of, LI-11, 118
arms and hands tired, GB-4, 224
arms and shoulders sore and painful, SI-11, 193
arms sore and weak, SI-10, 192
arms/back swollen and painful, TW-12, 187
arteriosclerosis, BL-62, 158; PC-8, 106
arthritis of the knee, BL-11, 82
arthritis of the leg and knee, GB-31, 162
ascites, CV-9, 54
asthma (chronic), KI-27, 203
asthma, BL-12, 83; CV-17, 43; CV-20, 170; CV-22, 42; CV-6, 58; GV-14, 74; LU-1, 47
asthma, such that the patient cannot sleep or sit, LV-14, 46
baby clenches teech, GB-37, 234
baby dies in the womb, SP-6, 134
baby moves in the uterus, SP-6, 134

Back

See also: pain of back, lumbago
backache with dyspnea, GB-25, 231
back cannot bend, BL-39, 241; BL-64, 24; BL-45, 243; GV-1, 808; BL-47, 97; GV-2, 79; KI-8, 146; SP-2, 132; BL-29, 240; GB-25, 231; BL-51, 244; ST-35, 221; BL-41, 242; SP-8, 205
back, carbuncle on, BL-12, 83
back cramped, LV-5, 211
back, difficult to bend, stretch, stand a long time, ST-37, 221
back, difficulty bending/straightening,
back, lower back pain, KI-12, 198
back pain, BL-44, 243; GB-20, 19; GV-2, 79; KI-8, 146; SP-8, 205
back pain (severe), BL-65, 249
back pain associated with constipation, SP-3, 204
back pain radiating to the lower abdomen, GB-29, 232
back stiff, BL-39, 241
bad temper, BL-18, 85
bedwetting, BL-25, 89; BL-27, 89; BL-28, 90; BL-54, 155; CV-4, 60; CV-6, 58; GV-2, 79; HT-5, 109; HT-7, 111; KI-2, 142; LV-1, 137; LV-2, 137; LV-3, 138; LV-9, 212; SP-6, 134; SP-9, 135
belching, CV-17, 43; HT-3, 108; KI-18, 200; KI-21, 201; LI-7, 180; LU-11, 102; LU-9, 101; PC-4, 103; PC-8, 106; ST-43, 223; XFi-2, 128
belching with pus, SP-20, 210
belching without appetite, TW-1, 121
Bells palsy, GB-13, 16
beri-beri, BL-57, 157; BL-60, 158; BL-61, 247; BL-63, 159; GB-39, 164; KI-8, 146; ST-3, 214; ST-32, 220; ST-33, 148; ST-35, 221; ST-37, 221; ST-39, 222; TW-10, 186; XFo-1, 165
beri-beri affecting the heart (severe), GB-31, 162
bitter taste in the mouth, BL-19, 85; GB-11, 227
BL-18, CV-1 and BL-23 for constant erection, CV-1, 62
BL-23 combined with LV-14 for painful intercourse, LV-14, 46
BL-31 location note, BL-34, 93
BL-32 location note, BL-34, 93
BL-33 location note, BL-34, 93
BL-34 location note, BL-34, 93
BL-38, treatment for weakness, BL-38, 95
BL-8 in combination with GV-4 for blindess, GV-4, 78

Bleeding

bleeding, excessive, LV-3, 138
bleeding, excessive after confinement, SP-6, 134
bleeding, excessive after confinement and patient is unconscious, TW-6, 123
bleeding, excessive after confinement with dizziness, HT-7, 111
bleeding excessive and dizziness, ST-36, 150
bleeding from the anus, LV-8, 139
bleeding from the nose, GV-23, 11
bleeding from the stomach, CV-12, 53
bleeding on the tongue, GB-11, 227
bleeding point, BL-2, 25; BL-54, 155; GV-15, 18; GV-25, 29; LU-11, 102; PC-9, 107; XF-2, 37; XF-6, 38; XF-7, 39; XH-3, 35
blockage of ear, SI-19, 22
blockage of nose, GV-22, 12
blood and semen in the urine, LU-7, 100
blood and/or pus in the stool, SP-16, 208
blood congested, KI-1, 141
blood in stools, GV-6, 171
blood in the urine, LI-8, 181; LU-9, 101
blood trapped in the uterus, SP-6, 134
blurred vision, KI-5, 196; TW-23, 26
body cannot turn, PC-8, 106
body chills/fevers, KI-19, 200
body feels heavy and joints are painful, SP-5, 133; SP-2, 132; SP-3, 204
body (whole) feels heavy, BL-58, 246
body fever (treats any), GV-14, 74
body fevers, BL-54, 155
body hair dry/rough, ST-39, 222
body is hot, patient is thirsty, PC-3, 103
body (whole) itching, LI-11, 118
body lazy, BL-43, 242
body numbness, LV-4, 138
body odor, HT-1, 177
body shaking, GB-38, 163
body weakness, LI-10, 117; BL-23, 88; BL-38, 95; XB-2, 97
body weakness with insomnia, BL-40, 241
body weakness with perspiration, BL-54, 155
bone cancer, SP-5, 133
bone, carbuncle on, GB-11, 227
borborygmi, BL-16, 239; BL-21, 86; BL-25, 89; BL-32, 91; BL-34, 92; BL-35, 93; BL-42, 242; BL-43, 242; BL-48, 244; GB-25, 231; GV-9, 77; KI-19, 200; KI-8, 146; LI-7, 180; LI-9, 181; SP-17, 208; SP-3, 204; SP-5, 133; SP-6, 134; SP-7, 204; ST-19, 217; ST-22, 218; ST-36, 150; ST-37, 221; ST-43, 223
borborygmi and full feelings in the abdomen, ST-20, 218
bowel incontinence, LI-10, 117
bowel movements, excessive, BL-41, 242; BL-42, 242; BL-43, 242
brain tumor, XH-2, 35
brain, weakness of, GB-20, 19
breach birth, BL-67, 159

Breast

See also: pain, swelling
breast abscess, LU-10, 176
breast cancer, CV-17, 43; GB-21, 71; SP-18, 46; ST-16, 45
breast carbuncle, GB-21, 71; GB-41, 234; GB-42, 235; KI-24, 202; LI-10, 117; LI-8, 181; SP-18, 46; ST-36, 150; ST-39, 222
breast carbuncle/tumor, KI-23, 201; ST-15, 217
breast disease, BL-46, 243
breast swollen and painful, CV-19, 169; ST-34, 220
breast ulcer or carbuncle,
breath difficult, SI-17, 195
breath, difficulty breathing deeply and talking, GV-14, 74
breath, difficulty in breathing during a fever, GB-21, 71
bronchitis, BL-12, 83; BL-13, 83; BL-17, 84; CV-19, 169; CV-22, 42; CV-23, 41; KI-24, 202; KI-25, 202; LU-3, 174
burning feeling in chest, ST-16, 45
calf cramping, GB-40, 164
calf pain, BL-58, 246; KI-9, 196

Cancer

See also: tumor
cancer, bone, SP-5, 133
cancer, breast, GB-21, 71; ST-16, 45
cancer of breast in the first stage, CV-17, 43

cancer, esophagus, CV-17, 43
cancer, stomach, BL-17, 84; BL-21, 86; CV-12, 53; SP-4, 133
cancers in the trunk, XB-1, 96
Following is a list of specific debilities. See also: indvidual body areas
cannot bear to wear clothes, HT-2, 177; SI-14, 186; ST-20, 218
cannot bend hips, BL-65, 249
cannot bend or straighten the knee, GB-33, 162; GB-34, 163
cannot breathe, KI-27, 203
cannot chew, GB-3, 224
cannot choose words, GV-20, 13
cannot close eyelid or blink, ST-4, 31
cannot close lips, LI-4, 115
cannot control the urine, GV-3, 79
cannot eat but likes to drink water, SP-20, 210
cannot eat or drink, BL-41, 242; BL-45, 243
cannot embrace, SI-13, 193
cannot lie down, GV-10, 77; TW-10, 186
cannot move arms, legs and torso tired TW-8, 185,
cannot move the four limbs, BL-59, 247; LI-13, 119
cannot move the toes after sitting, BL-58, 246,
cannot open the mouth, LU-7, 100; TW-6, 123
cannot raise the four limbs, LV-10, 212
cannot retract tongue, LI-7, 180
cannot sit or lie down, GV-2, 79
cannot straighten hand, HT-8, 112
cannot sleep or breathe, GB-23, 230
cannot speak, GB-20, 19; GV-15, 18; ST-6, 23; ST-4, 31
cannot speak or turn neck, SI-17, 195
cannot stand, XT-1, 153; BL-63, ST-36, 150; 159; GB-37, 234
cannot stand up after sitting down, GB-40, 164
cannot straighten the neck, GB-20, 19
cannot stretch, ST-31, 220
cannot swallow, LI-17, 183
cannot swallow food and liquids, CV-20, 170
cannot swallow liquids, CV-21, 170
cannot turn head, BL-37, 241; BL-65, 249; LI-15, 72; SI-16, 194
cannot walk, BL-60, 158
cannot walk/stand, LV-6, 211
carbuncle, BL-17, 84; GB-44, 165; PC-7, 105
carbuncle under the armpit, GB-22, 229; GB-41, 234

Cardiac

See also: heart, angina
cardiac diseases in general, GV-11, 76
cardiac pain, BL-16, 239; BL-64, 248; CV-14, 52; GV-8, 172; HT-1, 177; HT-3, 108; LU-4, 175; LU-8, 101; LU-9, 101; PC-2, 178; PC-5, 104
cardiac pain with the sensation of energy moving up, CV-11, 53
cardiomegaly, BL-17, 84; HT-7, 111; SI-1, 125
carditis, BL-13, 83; BL-15, 84; BL-17, 84; PC-5, 104
cataract, GB-3, 224; LI-1, 115; ST-3, 214; XFi-3, 128
catarrh from the bronchus, CV-23, 41
catarrh in the intestines, BL-20, 86
catarrh in the large intestine, BL-25, 89; BL-17, 84
catarrh in the stomach, BL-17, 84; BL-21, 86
catarrh of the bladder, ST-28, 67; LV-4, 138
cecum carbuncle, XA-2, 127
cerebral congestion, LI-1, 115; LU-11, 102; PC-9, 107
cerebral hemorrhage, GV-20, 13
cerebral weakness, CV-15, 51
cervical vertebrae, 3
chapped lips, LI-8, 181; ST-45, 153

Chest

See also: pain, swelling, inflammation
chest and abdomen swollen with gas, LV-14, 46
chest and back painful, LU-10, 176
chest and ribs full, KI-22, 201; KI-25, 202; SP-17, 208; SP-19, 209
chest and ribs painful, patient cannot lie down, LV-13, 48
chest and ribs swollen and painful, CV-16, 43
chest and ribs full with dyspnea, LI-5, 116; ST-13, 216; GB-40, 164
chest and upper abdomen problems, PC-6, 105

chest, burning sensation in the center of, XF-7, 39
chest feels hot and full with difficulty in breathing, ST-12, 45
chest, feeling of oppression and pain on, LU-2, 174
chest feels full, BL-53, 245; SP-20, 210; KI-23, 201; KI-27, 203
chest feels hot and painful, CV-13, 52
chest feels tight, GB-21, 71
chest feels uncomfortable, sad, BL-15, 84
chest full and painful, SP-18, 209; KI-24, 202
chest full and swollen, CV-20, 170; GB-35, 233
chest full with coughing and shortness of breath, CV-14, 52
chest full with coughing and vomiting, CV-15, 51
chest, hanging sensation under the chest, ST-26, 219
chest, melancholia, KI-24, 202
chest painful, CV-14, 52; CV-18, 169; GB-10, 227; GB-43, 235; KI-27, 203; SI-17, 195
chest painful, patient cannot turn their body, GB-43, 235
chest painful when coughing, GB-39, 164
chest, ribs and abdomen distended, SP-20, 210
chest suddenly feels full, GB-23, 230
chewing difficult, TW-20, 190

Chi

chi deficient, lack of energy of the whole body, CV-6, 58
chi disease, gastric pain, stomachache and not enough energy, CV-6, 58
chi felt rising up the chest, SP-15, 207; SP-18, 209; ST-30, 68; ST-37, 221; BL-16, 239
chi moving up, PC-8, 106; SP-10, 135; BL-38, 95 CV-18, 169; HT-9, 113; PC-1, 178; ST-10, 216; ST-20, 218
chi weak in the five viscera, CV-6, 58
child gets a headache from eating, BL-40, 241
child with cramping and stiffness who cannot drink milk, SI-5, 126
child with severe vomiting and diarrhea, SP-5, 133
childbirth, incessant bleeding, CV-5, 59
children crying at night, PC-9, 107
chilled feelings, ST-22, 218
chilled sensations below chest, KI-16, 199
chills, BL-45, 243; HT-2, 177
chills and fevers, BL-39, 241; KI-23, 201
cholera, BL-21, 86; CV-12, 53; CV-13, 52; CV-4, 60; CV-8, 55; HT-6, 110; LI-10, 117; LV-14, 46; PC-3, 103; PC-5, 104; SP-13, 206; SP-4, 133; SP-9, 135; ST-25, 66; ST-41, 151; ST-44, 152; ST-9, 215; TW-1, 121
cholera with cramping, BL-56, 246; BL-57, 157
cholera with vomiting, TW-6, 123
cholera with vomiting and diarrhea, BL-47, 97

Chronic

See also: individual disease entries
chronic asthma, KI-27, 203
chronic bleeding from the nose only, moxa, GV-23, 11
chronic chi disease, gastric pain, not enough energy, CV-6, 58
chronic constipation, TW-6, 123; XB-1, 96
chronic diarrhea, GV-20, 13; KI-12, 198; KI-13, 198
chronic dizziness (forehead), XH-4, 36
chronic hemorrhoids, BL-35, 93; BL-49, 244
chronic indigestion, XFi-1, 113
chronic indigestion in children, CV-5, 59; HT-8, 112
chronic inflammation of the testicles, XL-3, 157
chronic madness, ST-42, 152
chronic malaria, HT-8, 112; KI-6, 144; LV-13, 48
chronic piles, CV-1, 62
chronic sinusitis, GV-24, 11
chronic yawning in infants, TW-17, 22

Cold

See also: individual entries for each anatomical area
cold, GB-14, 25; GV-2, 79; LU-9, 101; LV-6, 211
cold/hot sensation, back, SI-15, 194
cold and hot sensations, GB-25, 231
cold chi rushing up to the chest, ST-41, 151
cold feeling starting at the shoulder and spreading, CV-6, 58; SI-14, 194

cold feeling around the umbilicus going up,
ST-25, 66
cold feeling ascending the four limbs, ST-44, 152
cold feeling in abdomen with cold sensations going up, CV-3, 61
cold feelings on the shins, LV-8, 139
cold feet, GB-35, 233
cold flu without fever, CV-6, 58
cold in the four limbs, GV-14, 74; CV-6, 58
cold in the scrotum, XSC-1, 63
cold on the back, BL-36, 240
cold sensation on the back preceding a high fever, BL-54, 155
cold sensation in the bones/marrow, LI-9, 181; ST-37, 221
cold sensation on arms, shoulders, chest or back, LU-7, 100
cold sensations, TW-10, 186
cold sensations from excessive drinking, LU-10, 176
cold sensations in the abdomen, CV-8, 55; SP-12, 206
cold sensations in the knee, ST-32, 220
cold sensations in the shins, ST-45, 153
cold sensations in the leg/tibia, LV-5, 211; ST-38, 222
cold sensations of the whole body, HT-6, 110
coldness and cramping of the four limbs, GV-4, 78
coldness in the four limbs because of the flu, LU-2, 174
coldness in the vagina and uterus, ST-28, 67
coldness, numbness of the whole leg and foot, GB-34, 163
coldness encroaching from foot to knee, KI-1, 141
colitis, LU-9, 101
color blindness, GB-1, 27
complete or partial loss of voice, GV-15, 18
conception difficult, CV-4, 60-61; KI-2, 142; KI-14, 198
confinement, LV-3, 138; SP-6, 134; ST-36, 150
confinement, no palpable pulse, LI-4, 115
congestion of brain, GV-20, 13; GV-21, 12; ST-8, 16
congestion of face, GV-21, 12; GV-22, 12; GV-23, 11
congestion of vagina, KI-2, 142
conjunctivitis, BL-1, 26; GB-1, 27; XF-4, 38; XHn-1, 129
conjunctivitis with film over the eve, LI-5, 116; SI-3, 125
constant erection, CV-1, 62
constipation, BL-25, 89; BL-27, 89; BL-28, 90; BL-30, 90; BL-31, 91; BL-32, 91; BL-33, 92; BL-34, 92; BL-49, 244; BL-56, 246; BL-57, 157; CV-12, 53; CV-6, 58; GB-34, 163; KI-15, 199; KI-16, 199; KI-18, 200; KI-3, 143; KI-4, 145; KI-6, 144; KI-7, 145; LV-1, 137; LV-13, 48; LV-2, 137; LV-3, 138; SP-2, 132; SP-5, 133; ST-36, 150; TW-6, 123; XB-1, 96
convergent strabismus, BL-2, 25
convulsions, GV-15, 18; GV-24, 11; GV-26, 31; GV-4, 78; TW-18, 189
convulsions and cramping, GV-1, 80
convulsions and cramping in children, SI-4, 126
convulsions in children, GB-13, 16; GB-15, 14; GB-4, 224; GV-11, 76; GV-12, 76; GV-20, 13; GV-21, 12; GV-22, 12; LI-16, 72; LU-7, 100; LV-1, 137; LV-2, 137; LV-3, 138; SI-1, 125; TW-23, 26; XF-3, 37

Cough

cough, dry, CV-22, 42
cough, hacking, CV-23, 41; ST-18, 46
coughing, BL-13, 83; BL-14, 238; BL-37, 241; BL-60, 158; CV-17, 43; CV-18, 169; CV-19, 169; CV-20, 170; CV-21, 170; GB-11, 227; GV-10, 77; GV-12, 76; GV-14, 74; KI-22, 201; KI-23, 201; KI-24, 202; KI-26, 202; KI-27, 203; KI-4, 145; LI-13, 119; LU-10, 176; LU-11, 102; LU-5, 99; LU-7, 100; LU-9, 101; PC-2, 178; SI-1, 125; SI-15, 194; SI-2, 191; SP-18, 209; SP-20, 210; SP-6, 134; ST-10, 216; ST-12, 45; ST-19, 217
coughing and a full feeling in the chest, LI-1, 115
coughing and cannot lie down, LU-1, 47
coughing and dyspnea, TW-10, 186; KI-25, 202; ST-14, 217; GB-44, 165
coughing, bouts of, LU-2, 174
coughing with a little blood, KI-1, 141
coughing with blood, GB-42, 235

coughing with chi rushing up, LU-8, 101; ST-13, 216; ST-15, 217
coughing with phlegm, GB-10, 227
coughing without appetite, KI-3, 143

Cramp

cramp on the arms, ST-32, 220
cramp of the arm (difficult to straighten), LI-10, 117
cramp in the upper abdominal region, CV-14, 52
cramp in the anus, BL-30, 90
cramp of the body, HT-4, 109; KI-1, 141
cramp in the calf, BL-52, 245
cramp on the chest, KI-24, 202
cramp in the diaphragm, CV-14, 52
cramp in the elbow, PC-7, 105; HT-8, 112; LI-11, 118; LI-5, 116; LU-5, 99; PC-5, 104; PC-6, 105
cramp of jaw, GB-2, 21; TW-17, 22
cramp of jaw after a stroke, ST-6, 23
cramp of knee (difficult to bend or stretch), LV-8, 139
cramp in the tongue, PC-9, 107
cramp in the stomach, CV-12, 53; BL-21, 86; BL-20, 86; BL-22, 87; ST-36, 150
cramp on the spine, BL-5, 236
cramp in the neck, BL-10, 18; GV-14, 74; SI-8, 127
cramp in the uterus, KI-4, 145; XT-1, 153; KI-1, 141
cramp of leg, BL-23, 88; ST-38, 222; GB-34, 163
cramp in lumbar area of back, ST-28, 67
cramp of scrotum such that the testicles are retracted, CV-5, 59
cramp of the penis, GV-1, 80; LV-1, 137
cramping, GV-4, 78; HT-4, 109; BL-67, 159; BL-8, 238
cramping and numbness of the face, XF-1, 36
cramping and twitching of eye or mouth, GV-26, 31
cramping and/or numbness of the five fingers, SI-4, 126
cramping from cholera, BL-52, 245; BL-59, 247; BL-61, 247; BL-63, 159; GB-34, 163; KI-1, 141; ST-18, 46
cramping in both legs and both legs without energy, BL-28, 90
cramping in children, LU-5, 99; PC-5, 104; BL-63, 159; SP-2, 132; TW-18, 189
cramping in part of the body, BL-63, 159
cramping in the back and in the knee, CV-7, 57
cramping of arm and elbow, SI-3, 125; TW-2, 121; TW-5, 123
cramping on the neck and shoulders, GV-13, 75
cramping with high fever, GV-12, 76
cramps and cold sensations, GB-25, 231
crazy (suddenly) like a ghost possessed the body, PC-5, 104
crazy laughing, ST-36, 150
crazy singing, ST-36, 150
crazy speech, LI-5, 116; LI-8, 181; ST-36, 150
crazy talking, KI-9, 196; LU-9, 101
cries easily, GB-24, 230; SP-14, 207
crying, HT-9, 113; KI-1, 141; ST-41, 151
crying (always) and frightened, PC-7, 105
crying and easily worried, GB-23, 230
crying at night, GV-20, 13; PC-5, 104
crying, excessive, HT-7, 111
crying, frequent, GV-20, 13
curved spine, XSP-1, 166
cutting pain in the abdomen, ST-40, 151; KI-16, 199
cutting pains below the navel, KI-14, 198
cutting pains when the abdomen is full, KI-17, 199
CV-1, BL-18 and BL-23 for constant erection, CV-1, 62
CV-3 treatment for weakness, BL-38, 95
CV-4 treatment for weakness, BL-38, 95
CV-6 treatment for weakness, BL-38, 95
CV-7 in combination with CV-9 for open fontanel, CV-7, 57
cystitis, CV-2, 62; BL-28, 90

Deafness

deafness, BL-23, 88; BL-63, 159; BL-65, 249; GB-10, 227; GB-2, 21; GB-3, 224; GB-43, 235; LI-1, 115; LI-4, 115; LI-5, 116; LI-6, 180; SI-1, 125; SI-16, 194; SI-17, 195; SI-19, 22; SI-3, 125; SI-8, 127; SI-9, 192; ST-1, 213; TW-10, 186; TW-17, 22; TW-2, 121; TW-21, 21; TW-3, 122; TW-5, 123; TW-7, 185; TW-8, 185; TW-9, 185
deafness (sudden), TW-16, 188
deafness, partial deafness, GB-20, 19; TW-16, 188
death, indications of ensuing death, KI-3, 143
death, point is forbidden for needle and moxa GV-17, 172

decay of the tongue with parched lips, LU-11, 102

Deep Needle Contraindicated

deep needle contraindicated, CV-14, 52; GB-21, 71; GB-3, 224; GB-4, 224; GB-5, 225; GV-15, 18; ST-2, 213; ST-9, 215
defecation, difficulty in passing urine and feces, ST-40, 151
defecation difficult, BL-50, 155; KI-1, 141; LV-4, 138
delirium, GV-12, 76; GV-16, 17; GV-26, 31; GV-27, 173; PC-5, 104; LU-7, 100
delirium with eyes looking left and right, SI-5, 126
dental abscess in gums, CV-24, 32
depression, GV-18, 172; LU-3, 174; TW-10, 186
depression of fontanel in child, GV-1, 80
diabetes, BL-23, 88; KI-2, 142; LV-1, 137; LV-2, 137; ST-33, 148
diaphragm cramping, BL-17, 84

Diarrhea

diarrhea, BL-21, 86; BL-25, 89; BL-26, 239; BL-32, 91; BL-33, 92; BL-34, 92; BL-35, 93; BL-44, 243; BL-65, 249; CV-12, 53; CV-4, 60; CV-5, 59; CV-8, 55; GB-25, 231; GV-1, 80; GV-20, 13; GV-4, 78; KI-12, 198; GV-5, 171;KI-13, 198; KI-16, 199; KI-21, 201; LI-3, 179; LV-13, 48; LV-14, 46; LV-3, 138; SP-1, 132; SP-14, 207; SP-5, 133; SP-9, 135; ST-22, 218; ST-36, 150; ST-37, 221; ST-44, 152; TW-18, 189
diarrhea with a lot of liquid, LV-8, 139
diarrhea with heavy feelings in the anus, KI-1, 141
diarrhea with pus and blood, ST-39, 222; SP-3, 204
diarrhea with pus and blood in female, KI-21, 201
diarrhea with swelling in abdomen and panting, ST-25, 66
diarrhea with undigested food, ST-21, 218

Difficulty

See also: cannot, specific anatomical areas
difficult for the patient to get up or bend, LV-5, 211
difficult to stand up, BL-62, 158; KI-2, 142; ST-34, 220
difficult to step on the floor, KI-1, 141; KI-2, 142; ST-39, 222
difficulty lifting the four limbs, PC-1, 178; LV-8, 139; SP-15, 207
difficulty lying down, SP-2, 132; SP-9, 135
difficulty lying down and turning the body from side to side, SP-19, 209
difficulty moving the lower leg, LV-5, 211
difficulty raising the arm/shoulder, GB-10, 227
difficulty sitting down, standing up, BL-62, 158; BL-58, 246; BL-59, 247
difficulty speaking, GV-9, 77; LI-11, 118; ST-36, 150
difficulty standing for a long time, BL-59, 247
difficulty walking, LV-4, 138
difficulty walking because of the legs, GB-10, 227
digestion, food and drink do not descend, BL-42, 242; BL-43, 242; CV-19, 169
digestion, food difficult to digest, CV-10, 54; CV-12, 53
digestion poor, BL-20, 86; CV-11, 53; ST-36, 150
dilatation of the heart, BL-16, 239
dilation of the stomach, CV-10, 54
discharge, See also: vaginal, red and white
discharge, XH-1, 34; CV-3, 61; CV-7, 57; CV-6, 58; XB-2, 97; BL-27, 89
discharge and/or dizziness after confinement, CV-7, 57
discharge, none after childbirth, CV-3, 61
discomfort in area of pharynx, LV-5, 211
disease of the gallbladder, BL-19, 85
disjointed, SP-21, 210
dislike of sunlight, ST-8, 16
dislikes wind and cold, GB-36, 233

Dizziness

dizziness, BL-11, 82; BL-6, 237; BL-62, 158; BL-8, 238; GB-20, 19; GV-20, 13; GV-21, 12; GV-24, 11; HT-5, 109; HT-6, 110; ST-36, 150; ST-8, 16; TW-23, 26; XF-3, 37; XH-2, 35; XH-3, 35
dizziness and fainting after needling, GV-26, 31
dizziness, forehead, XH-4, 36
dizziness from excessive uterine bleeding after childbirth, XF-3, 37
dizziness of the head, GV-4, 78
dizziness with vomiting, GV-24, 11
double tongue, CV-23, 41; GV-15, 18; LU-11, 102
dribbling after urination, KI-2, 142

dribbling of saliva, CV-23, 41; ST-39, 222
drop foot, BL-61, 247; GB-12, 228; GB-35, 233; GB-37, 234; GB-39, 164; ST-38, 222; ST-39, 222; ST-40, 151
dropping of eyelid, XF-4, 38
dropsy, CV-12, 53; CV-3, 61; KI-7, 145; SP-4, 133; KI-7, KI-8, 146; SP-8, 205; SP-9, 135; ST-36, 150; ST-44, 152; ST-45, 153
dropsy with swollen face, ST-43, 223
drowning, CV-1, 62
drunkenness, GB-8, 226
dumbness, CV-22, 42; CV-23, 41; CV-24, 32; ST-4, 31
during heavy winds the hair falls out of eyebrows, BL-54, 155
dysentery, CV-12, 53; KI-7, 145; ST-25, 66; BL-22, 87; BL-28, 90; CV-4, 60
dysentery in children, CV-8, 55
dysentery with pus and blood, BL-27, 89; LV-8, 139
dysmenorrhea, See also: menorrhalgia
dysmenorrhea, BL-23, 88; CV-3, 61; CV-4, 60; CV-6, 58; GB-26, 49; SP-10, 135
dysphonia, BL-11, 82

Dyspnea

dyspnea, BL-12, 83; BL-13, 83; BL-17, 84; BL-20, 86; BL-40, 241; BL-7, 237; CV-16, 43; CV-17, 43; CV-18, 169; CV-19, 169; CV-21, 170; CV-22, 42; CV-23, 41; CV-4, 60; GB-18, 228; GB-40, 164; GV-10, 77; GV-9, 77; KI-22, 201; KI-24, 202; KI-26, 202; LI-16, 72; LI-3, 179; LI-8, 181; LI-9, 181; LU-5, 99; LU-7, 100; SP-21, 210; ST-10, 216; ST-19, 217; ST-37, 221; TW-19, 189; LI-18, 183; LU-10, 176; LU-2, 174; LU-5, 99; SI-15, 194; ST-16, 45
dyspnea and difficulty talking, PC-5, 104
dyspnea and difficulty walking, GB-41, 234
dyspnea after lying down, BL-13, 83

Dysuria

See also: urination
dysuria, BL-26, 239; BL-49, 244; BL-50, 155; BL-67, 159; CV-3, 61; CV-4, 60; GB-25, 231; HT-8, 112; KI-1, 141; KI-10, 197; KI-7, 145; LV-10, 212; LV-2, 137; LV-3, 138; LV-4, 138; LV-5, 211; LV-9, 212; SP-6, 134; SP-7, 204; SP-8, 205; SP-9, 135
dysuria and difficulty defecating, GB-39, 164
dysuria and hematuria, BL-43, 242
ear, middle ear inflamed, TW-19, 189
ear swollen, TW-19, 189
eating difficulty, KI-21, 201
eats a lot but remains thin, BL-20, 86; BL-25, 89; SP-7, 204
eclampsia, GV-26, 31
edema, See also: swelling
edema, BL-20, 86; BL-23, 88; CV-7, 57; CV-8, 55; CV-9, 54; GB-28, 232; SP-6, 134
edema of face, GV-26, 31
edema of the whole body, ST-25, 66; ST-28, 67
eight liao points, BL-34, 93
ejaculation, weak force of, XSC-1, 63
elbow, difficult to bend, HT-9, 113; GB-44, 165
elbow or wrist, weakness in, LU-7, 100
emaciation, CV-6, 58; BL-21, 86; BL-22, 87; LI-15, 72; XB-2, 97
emaciation, body emaciated and feverish, GB-19, 229
emaciation due to TB, ST-36, 150
emaciation after intercourse during menstruation, CV-3, 61; SP-6, 134; BL-23, 88; CV-6, 58
emaciation (gradual), CV-10, 54; BL-38, 95; LI-10, 117; SP-6 135
emphysema, CV-17, 43; LU-5, 99; ST-16, 45
emphysema and numbness in the chest, LU-8, 101
enlargement of the liver, BL-18, 85
enlargement of the lungs, LU-9, 101
enlargement of the stomach, BL-21, 86; CV-12, 53; CV-9, 54
enteritis, BL-27, 89
epidemic, frog head epidemic, XH-3, 35; XF-6, 38
epigastrium swollen, KI-18, 200
epilepsy, BL-15, 84; BL-3, 236; BL-63, 159; CV-12, 53; CV-13, 52; CV-15, 51; GB-13, 16; GB-15, 14; GV-15, 18; GV-16, 17; GV-18, 172; GV-19, 13; GV-20, 13; GV-22, 12; GV-24, 11; GV-26, 31; GV-27, 173; GV-6, 171; GV-8, 172; HT-7, 111; KI-1, 141; PC-5, 104; PC-7, 105; PC-8, 106; SI-3, 125; SI-8, 127; SP-1, 132; SP-4, 133; TW-19, 189; TW-7, 185; XH-2, 35

epilepsy, during the daytime, BL-62, 158
epilepsy in children, BL-60, 158; CV-8, 55; GV-4, 78
epistaxis, BL-15, 84; BL-4, 236; BL-40, 241; BL-54, 155; BL-64, 248; BL-56, 246; BL-66, 249; BL-7, 237; GB-39, 164; GV-25, 29; GV-27, 173; HT-6, 110; HT-7, 111; KI-1, 141; LI-19, 184; LI-2, 179; LI-20, 29; LI-4, 115; LI-6, 180; LU-11, 102; LU-3, 174; LU-8, 101; LV-8, 139; PC-4, 103; SI-2, 191; SI-3, 125; ST-44, 152; ST-45, 153; TW-10, 186
eruptions, ST-32, 220
esophageal spasm, CV-22, 42
excess saliva, SI-17, 195
excess tearing, BL-65, 249
excessive bleeding after labor with dizziness, PC-6, 105
excessive secretion on the part of the female, BL-23, 88; ST-30, 68
excessive sleep, KI-4, 145; LV-1, 137
external swelling of the throat, TW-2, 121

Eye

See also: pain, vision, inflammation
eye, BL-8 in combination with GV-4 for blindess, GV-4, 78
eye, blindness (sudden), GV-4, 78
eyes, blinking of, ST-8, 16
eyes, congestion of outer corners, GB-15, 14
eyes, rolling of, GV-8, 172
eyes, dizziness/pain in, BL-58, 246; GB-17, 228
eye dimness, BL-4, 236; GB-44, 165; BL-23, 88; GB-4, 224; LI-13, 119; ST-36, 150; XH-3, 35
eye diseases, BL-1, 26; BL-18, 85; GB-37, 234
eye dizziness, BL-1, 26; BL-3, 236; BL-64, 248; GB-13, 16; GB-20, 19; GB-41, 234; BL-5, 236; BL-66, 249; BL-65, 249; GV-4, 78; BL-11, 82; LU-10, 176; HT-5, 109; LU-3, 174; SI-5, 126; SP-2, 132; ST-41, 151; TW-3, 122; ST-2, 213
eye red and feels rough, TW-2, 121
eye wanders, BL-2, 25
eyes dim from overeating spicy foods, BL-18, 85
eyes, film on, BL-6, 237; BL-67, 159; GB-15, 14; TW-1, 121; TW-20, 190; TW-3, 122; XFi-3, 128; GV-28, 173
eyes, film on (beginning), XH-1, 34
eyes fixed upwards, GV-8, 172
eyes as if smoke is inside, ST-2, 213
eyes, inflamation, BL-2, 25
eyes itching, ST-2, 213
eyes jaundiced, HT-9, 113; HT-2, 177; BL-65, 249; SI-18, 195
eyes locked looking up, BL-5, 236; GB-14, 25; ST-1, 213; TW-23, 26
eyes red and painful, ST-1, 213; ST-2, 213
eyes red and painful, with headache, BL-2, 25
eyes red and swollen, GB-14, 25
eyes red, swollen and painful, TW-23, 26
eyes red/painful from inner canthus, KI-11, 197; KI-12, 198; KI-13, 198; KI-14, 198; KI-17, 199; KI-18, 200
eyes twitch, GB-14, 25; SI-18, 195
eyes twitching or blinking separately, TW-23, 26
eyes weepy, GV-24, 11
eyes weepy and dizzy, BL-18, 85
eyes with cold sensations and tears, ST-1, 213
eyes, yellow matter in, TW-18, 189
eyelid dropping down, BL-1, 26
eyelids with heavy feeling, GB-19, 229
eyesight, deterioration of, BL-2, 25; GV-7, 171
eyesight poor, BL-21, 86; GV-26, 31; HT-1, 177

Face

See also: pain; swelling, inflammation
face feels cold, without perspiration, GV-23, 11
face feels hot, CV-22, 42
face hot, without perspiration, HT-5, 109
face, one side paralyzed, GB-3, 224; ST-42, 152;
ST-45, 153
face pale, GV-22, 12
face paralyzed, LI-10, 117
face paralyzed causing dimness of the eyes, GB-7, 226
face red and swollen, GB-6, 225; GV-23, 11
face swollen, GB-35, 233; GB-5, 225; SP-4, 133; ST-5, 214
face swollen, pale and yellow, TW-16, 188
face twisted, ST-1, 213
facial paralysis, BL-6, 237; BL-7, 237; GB-12, 228; LU-7, 100; SI-18, 195; LI-2, 179; ST-3, 214; ST-5, 214; ST-7, 215; ST-8, 16; TW-23, 26

facial paralysis and muteness, ST-2, 213
facial spasm, ST-3, 214; TW-22, 190
fainting, GV-26, 31; LU-7, 100
fainting, patient cannot talk, death-like, ST-45, 153
fainting with a darkened face, KI-1, 141
fainting without sensation, CV-3, 61
faints suddenly as if dying, LV-1, 137
false call to stool, GB-27, 231
false urge to bowel movement due to pelvic pressure, GB-26, 49
fear, GV-16, 17
fear and forgetfulness, GV-20, 13
fear of cold winds, GB-3, 224; PC-2, 178; TW-22, 190; GB-18, 228
fear of people, HT-8, 112; PC-4, 103
fear of wind and cold, GV-19, 13; BL-44, 243
feces too dry, BL-46, 243; BL-52, 245
feeling of hatred for human noise, CV-15, 51
feet cold, LV-3, 138
feet swollen, BL-27, 89
female sterility, KI-18, 200
fetus dies in uterus, XT-1, 153

Fever

fever, See also: High fever, Intermittent fever
fever, PC-1, 178; BL-53, 245; GV-16, 17; LI-6, 180; SP-3, 204
fever (severe), GV-4, 78; XFi-4, 129
fever and chills, GB-16, 14; BL-59, 247
fever and chills similar to malaria, PC-1, 178
fever and headache, LI-7, 180
fever starting in the afternoon, LU-5, 99
fever with sensations of cold, ST-16, 45
fever with shivering, BL-16, 239
fever without perspiration, BL-4, 236; BL-40, 241; GB-16, 14; GB-5, 225
fibroids below navel make an upturned cup, CV-4, 60
fibula painful, GB-37, 234
fingers cannot clench, LU-6, 175
fingers, difficulty in bending or moving the five fingers, LI-4, 115; TW-3, 122
fingers numb and cramped, PC-7, 105
fingers numb and painful, XHn-1, 129
flatulence, BL-21, 86; SP-7, 204

Flu

See also: fever, high fever, intermittent fever
flu, GV-16, 17; SI-9, 192; KI-3, 143
flu, a feeling of overheating, LV-14, 46
flu, beginning of, feels cold with fever, GB-20, 19
flu, encroaching cold, SP-2, 132
flu, four limbs hot after the flu, GV-2, 79; BL-54, 155
flu, high fever without perspiration and cold sensations, BL-11, 82
flu, hot sensations in the stomach, ST-39, 222
flu, the chest feels hot, PC-5, 104
flu with a high fever and no perspiration, LU-8, 101; LI-1, 115; GB-43, 235; KI-8, 146; LU-10, 176
flu with excessive thirst, LI-4, 115
flu with high temperature and cold sensations, GV-14, 74
flu with hot sensations, LI-3, 179
fluid coming from the ear, TW-21, 21
fontanel does not close in child, CV-9, 54
foolishness, CV-15, 51; HT-7, 111; KI-4, 145
foot and toes stiff, XFo-1, 165
foot inflamed, XFo-1, 165
foot swollen, BL-60, 158; KI-6, 144; XFo-1, 165
forearm cold, difficult to raise, HT-1, 177
forehead headache, GB-13, 16
forehead pain, BL-63, 159
forgetfulness, BL-15, 84; BL-38, 95; GV-11, 76; LU-7, 100; HT-3, 108; HT-7, 111; KI-21, 201

Four Limbs

See also: arms, legs, pain, swelling, inflammation
four limbs cold, PC-5, 104
four limbs cramped, GB-11, 227
four limbs immobile, SP-14, 207
four limbs lazy and tired, KI-6, 144
four limbs swollen, GV-9, 77; LI-7, 180; SP-2, 132
four limbs tired, LV-13, 48; PC-7, 105
four limbs tired and cold, SP-6, 134
four limbs weak, CV-6, 58; GB-23, 230; SI-7, 192

four limbs, cold encroaching, LV-2, 137
fright, excessive, ST-45, 153
frightened, GV-24, 11; BL-64, 248; GB-9, 226; HT-7, 111; HT-9, 113; LU-10, 176; PC-5, 104; ST-36, 150
frightened and cannot sleep, CV-6, 58
frightened and lacks chi, LV-3, 138
frightened and unhappy, KI-4, 145; LV-5, 211
frightened easilly, PC-3, 103
frightened, fearful of being captured, KI-1, 141; KI-2, 142
frightened in the heart, BL-15, 84
frightened, worried, insane, SI-7, 192

Full Feeling

See also: abdomen, pain
full feeling in abdomen, BL-40, 241
full feeling in chest, LU-2, 174; CV-18, 169; HT-1, 177; PC-1, 178; GB-36, 233; BL-14, 238; GB-41, 234; PC-2, 178;
full feeling in chest and abdomen, KI-1, 141
full feeling in chest and abdomen with vomiting, SP-2, 132
full feeling in chest and sides of body, ST-14, 217; KI-26, 202
full feeling in chest with pain, ST-18, 46
full feeling in lower abdomen, LI-8, 181
full feeling in lungs, KI-19, 200
full feeling in stomach with vomiting, ST-25, 66; TW-15, 188
full feeling in the chest with the chi rushing, BL-39, 241
full feeling in the chest with weakness, GB-22, 229
full feeling in the lower abdomen, KI-21, 201; LV-10, 212
full feeling in the upper abdomen, ST-19, 217; ST-22, 218
full feeling on the chest and loins, PC-8, 106
full feeling under the chest, KI-20, 200; LI-13, 119
furuncle, GV-10, 77; GV-12, 76; XA-2, 127
furuncle on lips, XF-6, 38
gallbladder stone or kidney stone, XB-1, 96

Gas

gas, enlargement of abdomen, SP-4, 133; SP-5, 133
gas, enlargement of stomach, CV-13, 52; SP-6, 134
gas, feeling of gas ascending from the lower abdomen, CV-7, 57
gas, from stomach rising up, ST-36, 150
gas in abdomen, BL-28, 90; LV-13, 48
gas in intestines, LI-9, 181
gas in lower abdomen moving up and down, ST-29, 68; KI-13, 198
gas, like a stone in the abdomen but moving, BL-26, 239
gas lump inside abdomen, KI-1, 141
gas moving in the abdomen, KI-14, 198; ST-19, 217
gas moving up and down in abdomen, KI-12, 198
gas in abdomen causing pain at the umbilicus, ST-22, 218
gas stagnant in the lower abdomen (like a stone), LV-5, 211
gas under ribs at the sides of body, LV-14, 46; ST-21, 218
gastric hemorrhage, BL-21, 86
gastric pain, BL-43, 242; CV-15, 51; KI-18, 200; SP-2, 132; ST-43, 223
gastric pain (severe), SP-5, 133
gastric spasm, CV-10, 54
gastritis, BL-21, 86; CV-10, 54
gastroenteritis, CV-12, 53
gastroptosis, CV-8, 55
GB-2 combined with PC-5 TW-17 LI-4 GV-20 for muteness, GV-15, 18
GB-43 one of the eight winds, XFo-1, 165
gingivitis, GV-27, 173
gingivitis in children, PC-8, 106
glossitis, LI-7, 180
glottis spasm, CV-22, 42
goiter, BL-7, 237; CV-22, 42; ST-11, 216; TW-13, 187; XN-1, 34
gonorrhea, BL-15, 84; BL-23, 88; BL-27, 89; BL-32, 91; BL-57, 157; CV-2, 62; CV-3, 61; CV-5, 59; GV-1, 80; KI-11, 197; KI-2, 142; KI-4, 145; KI-7, 145; LV-1, 137; LV-4, 138; SP-10, 135; SP-6, 134; ST-36, 150
gonorrhea in males, SP-11, 205
gums swollen, GB-9, 226; ST-7, 215; TW-20, 190

GV-20 combined with PC-5, TW-17, LI-4, GB-2 for muteness, GV-15, 18
GV-26 in combination with LI-20 for numbness and itching, LI-20, 29
GV-4 in combination with BL-18 for blindness, GV-4, 78
hair dropping out, GV-20, 13
hair gray at a youthful age, GV-20, 13
halitosis, GV-27, 173; GV-28, 173; PC-7, 105; PC-8, 106
hallucinations, GV-16, 17; BL-2, 25
hands and feet hot without perspiration, GB-44, 165
hatred of human voices, ST-44, 152
hatred of the wind, BL-65, 249
hay fever, BL-2, 25
head, SP-4, 133
head tilted up, BL-5, 236

Headache

See also: migraine
head feels like its going to explode, PC-9, 107; KI-1, 141
head heavy and painful, BL-59, 247
headache, BL-11, 82; BL-19, 85; BL-3, 236; BL-6, 237; BL-62, 158; BL-67, 159; GB-1, 27; GB-12, 228; GB-16, 14; GB-5, 225; GV-15, 18; GV-16, 17; GV-20, 13; GV-21, 12; HT-2, 177; HT-3, 108; HT-5, 109; HT-6, 110; LI-4, 115; LI-5, 116; LU-6, 175; PC-1, 178; SI-1, 125; SI-4, 126; ST-2, 213; ST-36, 150; ST-40, 151; ST-41, 151; TW-1, 121; TW-12, 187; TW-2, 121; TW-22, 190; TW-3, 122; XF-3, 37; XHn-1, 129
headache (severe), ST-8, 16; BL-64, 248; BL-9, 238; GV-18, 172; GV-4, 78; KI-1, 141; PC-9, 107
headache (severe) on top of the head with dizziness, BL-60, 158
headache (severe) with heavy feelings on one side, GB-19, 229
headache and epistaxis associated with malaria, BL-58, 246
headache and eyes dizzy with the flu, BL-22, 87
headache and neck stiff, TW-20, 190
headache (forehead), XH-4, 36; GB-14, 25; GV-23, 11; GV-24, 11
headache in whole head and/or occipital region, GB-20, 19
headache on one side of the head, GB-7, 226; GB-8, 226
headache on the top of the head, BL-4, 236; GB-18, 228; GB-21, 71
headache radiating to the jaw and neck, BL-65, 249
headache with fever, BL-23, 88; TW-19, 189
headache with melancholia, GB-44, 165
headaches, temple, TW-23, 26
headache (occipital), GV-19, 13
heart and chest painful, CV-17, 43
heart and stomach painful, CV-12, 53
heart, burning sensation in chest or heart, CV-1, 62
heart painful as if it had been stabbed, KI-2, 142
heart palpitations, BL-15, 84; GB-19, 229; HT-9, 113; KI-1, 141; PC-5, 104
heart suspended as though hungry, PC-7, 105
heart weakness, GV-20, 13; PC-5, 104
heat stroke, GV-26, 31
heavy feeling in anus after bowel movement, ST-41, 151
heavy feeling in the head, BL-10, 18; BL-7, 237; GV-20, 13; BL-66, 249; ST-32, 220
heavy feeling of the eyelids, BL-10, 18; LV-2, 137
heavy feelings in the head with leg cramps, BL-54, 155
heavy feelings in the legs, ST-39, 222
heavy feelings in the lumbar area, BL-54, 155
heel pain, BL-56, 246; BL-57, 157; BL-61, 247; ST-39, 222
hematemesis, See also: vomiting
hematemesis, BL-15, 84; BL-18, 85; CV-17, 43; LU-9, 101
BL-38, 95; HT-6, 110; LU-5, 99; SI-2, 191
hematuria, See also: urine, urination
hematuria, BL-23, 88; BL-32, 91; CV-4, 60 CV-3, 61; CV-6, 58; LI-8, 181; PC-7, 105
hematuria and blood in feces, PC-8, 106
hemiplegia, GB-30, 161; GB-34, 163; GV-20, 13; LI-15, 72; LI-9, 181; LU-7, 100; ST-8, 16
hemiplegia and cannot lie on one side, BL-15, 84
hemiplegia following a stroke, LI-11, 118; GB-39, 164

hemoptysis, CV-15, 51; CV-17, 43; BL-13, 83; BL-15, 84; BL-18, 85; BL-38, 95; CV-18, 169; CV-22, 42; HT-7, 111; KI-2, 142; LI-13, 119; LU-10, 176; LU-5, 99; LU-6, 175; LU-9, 101; LV-2, 137; LV-3, 138; PC-3, 103; PC-7, 105; SI-15, 194
hemorrhage of intestines, BL-17, 84; BL-35, 93
hemorrhage of the mouth, LU-11, 102
hemorrhage of the rectum, BL-25, 89; BL-51, 244; GV-1, 80
hemorrhage of the uterus, CV-5, 59; CV-2, 62; LV-2, 137; SP-2, 132
hemorrhaging of uterus (severe), SP-1, 132; SP-6, 134; LV-1, 137
hemorrhage of the vagina, CV-3, 61
hemorrhage of the womb, CV-6, 58
hemorrhoids, See also: piles
hemorrhoids, BL-24, 239; BL-27, 89; BL-35, 93; BL-49, 244; BL-56, 246; BL-65, 249; GV-6, 171
hemorrhoids and bleeding of the rectum, GV-4, 78
hemorrhoids painful/swollen, BL-58, 246
hemorrhiods with ulcers, XB-2, 97
hepatitis, LV-13, 48; LV-14, 46; ST-45, 153
hepatomegaly, BL-21, 86; BL-23, 88
hernia, BL-55, 245; BL-63, 159; CV-14, 52; CV-3, 61; CV-4, 60; GB-40, 164; GV-1, 80; KI-1, 141; KI-6, 144; LV-1, 137; LV-2, 137; LV-3, 138; SP-13, 206; ST-27, 67; ST-29, 68; ST-36, 150; XL-3, 157; XT-1, 153
hernia and/or pain, inflammation in testicle, CV-6, 58
hernia below the navel, KI-14, 198
hernia in a child, KI-9, 196
hiccoughs, ST-18, 46; TW-17, 22; CV-22, 42; KI-3, 143; XFi-2, 128
hiccoughs (severe), XT-1, 153
high blood pressure, ST-36, 150

High Fever

See also: fever, intermittent fever
high fever and no sweating, SI-1, 125
high fever for several days without perspiration, PC-8, 106
high fever with chills and no perspiration, ST-43, 223
high fever with cold sensations, flu, GV-13, 75; SI-9, 192
high fever with headache, PC-7, 105; LU-10, 176
high fever without perspiration, LI-11, 118; TW-10, 186; BL-54, 155; GB-37, 234; GB-6, 225; KI-3, 143; LU-6, 175; PC-9, 107; SI-2, 191; SI-4, 126; SI-5, 126; SP-2, 132; ST-45, 153; TW-1, 121; TW-3, 122; TW-6, 123
high fever with burning sensation, PC-9, 107
high fever with full feeling in chest, HT-9, 113
high fever with melancholia in the heart, LI-5, 116
homicidal mania, GV-12, 76

Hot

hot and cold feelings, SI-10, 192
hot feeling below umbilicus, CV-7, 57
hot feeling in the chest, BL-12, 83; KI-1, 141; SP-1, 132; ST-36, 150
hot feeling in the chest during the flu, LU-1, 47
hot feeling in the four limbs, LI-15, 72
hot feelings in the whole chest, BL-11, 82
hot sensation in the lower abdomen, KI-15, 199; GB-23, 230
hot sensations, GB-24, 230; LV-10, 212
hot sensations and itching skin on the palms, PC-8, 106
hot sensation on the palms, LU-9, 101; HT-8, 112; PC-7, 105; LU-8, 101; LU-11, 102; PC-5, 104
hot sensations from urination, BL-52, 245
hot sensations in shoulders, or finger and small finger, ST-39, 222
hot sensations in the head, BL-5, 236
hot sensations in the inner thigh, BL-55, 245
hot sensations in the leg, cannot stand, ST-38, 222
hot sensations in the mouth, KI-4, 145
hot sensations in the stomach, GB-39, 164; ST-37, 221
hot sensations of the sole, BL-67, 159; KI-1, 141
hot sensations on hands and feet without perspiration, GB-11, 227
hot sensations on the face, ST-39, 222
hot sensations on the shoulder above the clavicle, SI-9, 192

HT-3 and ST-33 for Parkinsons disease, ST-33, 148
HT-9 with LV-2 for vaginal odors, HT-9, 113
hunchback, BL-13, 83
hunchback with the sternum also protruding, GB-36, 233
hunger, excessive, ST-45, 153
hungry without appetite, CV-3, 61
hypertension, PC-8, 106; PC-9, 107; SP-1, 132; SP-6, 134
hysteria, GV-14, 74; GV-26, 31
impotence, BL-15, 84; BL-23, 88; CV-3, 61; CV-4, 60; GV-4, 78; KI-10, 197
incontinence of urine, GV-4, 78; LU-10, 176; SP-11, 205; ST-22, 218
indigestion, BL-21, 86; BL-47, 97; BL-48, 244; BL-66, 249; CV-13, 52; GV-5, 171; KI-20, 200; LV-13, 48; SP-13, 206; SP-16, 208; SP-3, 204; SP-5, 133; SP-7, 204; SP-9, 135; XFi-1, 113
indigestion in children, CV-5, 59; HT-8, 112
indigestion in large intestine, ST-37, 221

Inflammation

See also: swelling, pain
inflammation and pain in the eyes, GB-16, 14
inflammation, general, XA-2, 127
inflammation of arm, XHn-1, 129
inflammation of breast glands, GB-21, 71; KI-24, 202
inflammation of cecum, BL-25, 89; CV-5, 59; XA-1, 104; XA-2, 127
inflammation of ear, SI-19, 22; TW-21, 21
inflammation of elbow, LI-11, 118
inflammation of eyeball and film over iris, BL-18, 85
inflammation of eyes, ST-8, 16; PC-6, 105; XF-2, 37; GB-20, 19
inflammation of hip joint, GB-30, 161
inflammation of kidneys, BL-22, 87; BL-47, 97; BL-23, 88; BL-25, 89
inflammation of knee, XL-1, 148
inflammation of the knee, crane knee, GB-34, 163
inflammation and/or swelling of the knee, GB-33, 162
inflammation of larynx and pharynx, KI-2, 142
inflammation of middle ear, GB-2, 21; ST-7, 215
inflammation of mouth, BL-13, 83
inflammation of ovaries, ST-30, 68; ST-29, 68
inflammation of rectum, GV-1, 80
inflammation or pain in testicles, CV-3, 61; BL-33, 92
inflammation of testicles, SP-6, 134; BL-31, 91; BL-32, 91; CV-4, 60; KI-2, 142; ST-28, 67; ST-30, 68; LV-1, 137; ST-29, 68
inflammation of otitis media, LI-4, 115
inflammation of pericardium, PC-9, 107; CV-15, 51
inflammation of rectum, BL-26, 239
inflammation of spine, KI-8, 146
inflammation of stomach, CV-12, 53
inflammation of throat, ST-12, 45
inflammation of uterus, CV-2, 62
inflammation of uterus metritis, BL-28, 90
inflammation of vagina, SP-9, 135
inflammed, swollen, infected ovaries, BL-31, 91
inguinal adenitis, SP-11, 205
inner canthus, See also: eyes
inner canthus painful, BL-67, 159
inner canthus red/painful, BL-1, 26; BL-64, 248; BL-65, 249; KI-15, 199; KI-16, 199; KI-19, 200; KI-20, 200; KI-21, 201
inner foot pain, SP-5, 133
insanity, GB-12, 228; GB-36, 233; GB-37, 234; GB-9, 226; GV-18, 172; GV-27, 173; GV-6, 171; GV-8, 172; KI-20, 200; LI-7, 180; XH-2, 35
insanity (not severe), GV-20, 13
insanity with hallucinations, BL-61, 247
insanity with total body cramping, BL-5, 236
insomnia, BL-13, 83; HT-7, 111; LU-9, 101; SI-1, 125; SP-1, 132; SP-6, 134; SP-9, 135
insomnia caused by fright, ST-27, 67
insuring long life, ST-36, 150
intercostal neuralgia, GB-11, 227; GB-34, 163; KI-25, 202; KI-26, 202; LV-14, 46; ST-16, 45; TW-6, 123
intercostal pain, BL-18, 85; HT-2, 177
intercostal pain and numbness, ST-18, 46
intermittent fever, BL-19, 85
intermittent fevers and chills, LI-4, 115
intestinal hemorrhage, BL-34, 92; SP-4, 133

intestinal pain, LV-1, 137; LV-2, 137; SP-6, 134; ST-22, 218
intestines with cold sensations, BL-29, 240
iris, film on, GB-40, 164; LI-4, 115
iris, white spot covering the pupil, BL-64, 248; ST-3, 214; TW-23, 26

Itching

itching, LI-11, 118; LI-4, 115; LI-5, 116; SP-10, 135; ST-32, 220; TW-6, 123
itching eruptions on the skin, LI-11, 118
itching in anus, pruritis ani, CV-1, 62
itching in eyes, BL-2, 25; GB-14, 25; XFi-3, 128; ST-1, 213; ST-4, 31
itching on eyelids, LI-3, 179
itching on face, LI-20, 29
itching on palm, XHn-1, 129
itching or numbness of the whole body, GB-31, 162
itching in the scrotum, LV-5, 211; SP-10, 135
itching in the vagina, CV-3, 61; CV-7, 57; HT-8, 112; KI-6, 144; LV-8, 139; KI-2, 142
itching sores, BL-17, 84

Jaundice

jaundice, BL-12, 83; BL-15, 84; BL-18, 85; BL-19, 85; BL-20, 86; BL-21, 86; CV-12, 53; CV-13, 52; CV-14, 52; GV-16, 17; GV-28, 173; GV-6, 171; GV-9, 77; HT-7, 111; KI-1, 141; LI-2, 179; PC-6, 105; PC-8, 106; SI-3, 125; SI-4, 126; SP-5, 133
jaundice and fever, BL-44, 243
jaundice with yellow eyes, HT-1, 177; SI-8, 127
jaw, ST-7, 215
jaw cramp, GB-3, 224
jaw cramped and swollen, GB-12, 228
jaw stiff, TW-22, 190
jaw swollen, GB-43, 235; SI-11, 193; SI-16, 194
jaw swollen, toothache, ST-5, 214
jaw swollen without toothache, SI-18, 195
joints, SP-21, 210
keratitis, GB-1, 27
KI-7 with KI-8 for dropsy, KI-8, 146
KI-7 with LI-4 and PC-5 to revive the pulse, LI-4, 115
KI-8 with LI-4 and PC-5 for cessation of the pulse, KI-8, 146
kidney stone or gallbladder stone, XB-1, 96
kidneys weak, BL-29, 240
kidneys, weakness of, with lumbar ache, BL-23, 88; GV-4, 78

Knee

See also: pain, swelling, inflammation
knee and leg weakness, XL-2, 149
knee and shin cramps, ST-41, 151
knee cannot be bent or stretched, KI-10, 197
knee inflammation, GB-38, 163; SP-9, 135
knee pain, BL-54, 155; GB-35, 233; GB-37, 234; LV-2, 137; LV-7, 139; ST-38, 222; ST-45, 153
knee swollen, BL-61, 247; ST-3, 214; ST-37, 221
knees and feet cold like ice, BL-23, 88
knees, hardness behind the knees, BL-60, 158
knees with cold sensations, BL-32, 91
labor difficult, BL-60, 158; GB-21, 71; LV-14, 46; SP-6, 134; ST-30, 68
lack of spirit, HT-7, 111
lack of yang and weakness of the whole body, CV-3, 61
lack of yin with headaches, CV-1, 62
lacks energy, SP-21, 210
lacrymation, See also: tearing
lacrymation excessive, XFi-3, 128
lactation, CV-8, 55
lactation insufficient, ST-18, 46; SI-1, 125; SI-2, 191; SP-12, 206; CV-17, 43; PC-1, 178
laryngitis, ST-4, 31
laughter, LU-7, 100; LI-5, 116; PC-7, 105
laughter excessive, HT-7, 111; ST-40, 151
laziness, ST-40, 151
lazy and sleepy, SP-5, 133

Leg

See also: pain, inflammation, swelling; four limbs
leg and arm cramps, LI-1, 115
leg and foot cramps, GB-39, 164
leg cold/numb, ST-39, 222; ST-34, 220; GB-32, 232; GB-38, 163
leg cramps, GB-44, 165; BL-64, 248

leg numb and becoming withered, BL-59, 247
leg stiffness, GB-38, 163; BL-56, 246
leg weakness, BL-10, 18; ST-33, 148; BL-54, 155; ST-39, 222
leukorrhea, BL-27, 89; CV-3, 61; ST-25, 66
leukorrhea and gonorrhea, CV-4, 60
LI-11 combination with LI-4, PC-9 for double tongue, GV-15, 18
LI-4 combined with PC-5, TW-17, GB-2, GV-20 for muteness, GV-15, 18
LI-4 with KI-7 and PC-5 to revive the pulse, LI-4, 115
LI-4 with KI-8 and PC-5 for cessation of the pulse, KI-8, 146
limbs, See also: four limbs, legs, arms
limbs weak, ST-27, 67; GB-24, 230
lin chi, GB-15 as measure for XH-3, XH-3, 35
lips dry, ST-39, 222
lips stiff, GB-17, 228; TW-20, 190; TW-21, 21
lips swollen, LV-3, 138
lips trembling, ST-5, 214
lips/jaws swollen/painful, ST-3, 214
lively dreams, TW-16, 188
local hernia, XSC-1, 63
lockjaw, CV-24, 32; PC-9, 107; ST-4, 31
lockjaw in children, BL-57, 157
loosening of energy on the spine, BL-64, 248

Lower abdomen

See also: abdomen, pain, inflammation, swelling
lower abdomen, GB-24, 230
lower abdomen cramp, GB-25, 231; BL-63, 159
lower abdomen hard, ST-36, 150
LU-11 in combination with TW-5 for weakness of hand, TW-5, 123

Lumbago

See also: back, pain, spine, sciatica
lumbago, BL-24, 239; BL-26, 239; BL-29, 240; BL-49, 244; BL-56, 246; BL-57, 157; BL-59, 247; BL-28, 90; BL-62, 158; BL-64, 248; GB-31, 162; GB-34, 163; GB-38, 163; GB-39, 164; GV-26, 31; GV-3, 79; KI-1, 141; KI-3, 143; LV-2, 137; SP-2, 132; SP-9, 135; ST-31, 220; ST-36, 150; TW-10, 186
lumbago reacting to the knee, GB-30, 161
lumbar ache, BL-25, 89; GB-25, 231; XB-2, 97
lumbar and thigh painful, GB-40, 164
lumbar area cold and sore as if sitting in cold water, GB-38, 163
lumbar area cold like ice, BL-23, 88
lumbar area stiff, GV-1, 80
lumbar pain, GV-2, 79
lumbar, thigh, knees are cold like water, numb, ST-33, 148
lumbar vertebrae, 3
lump below navel sometimes moving, CV-3, 61
lumps or abscess on the neck, SI-17, 195
lung congestion, CV-16, 43
lungs withered, overcooled, BL-37, 241
lungs withering, BL-13, 83
lust, SP-20, 210
LV-2 one of the eight winds, XFo-1, 165
mad speech, LI-6, 180
mad speech and patient unhappy, PC-7, 105
madness, BL-11, 82; BL-15, 84; BL-2, 25; BL-57, 157; BL-58, 246; BL-62, 158; BL-65, 249; CV-14, 52; CV-15, 51; GB-13, 16; GV-1, 80; GV-24, 11; GV-26, 31; KI-9, 196; LI-6, 180; SI-3, 125; SI-5, 126; ST-24, 219; ST-40, 151; ST-41, 151; ST-42, 152; ST-45, 153; TW-12, 187
madness (sudden), PC-5, 104; XFi-4, 129
madness and fearfulness with delirium and nonsensical speech, ST-39, 222
madness with cramping, LI-11, 118
madness with patient running arond crazily, SI-8, 127

Malaria

malaria, BL-11, 82; BL-20, 86; BL-38, 95; BL-40, 241; BL-57, 157; BL-63, 159; BL-64, 248; GB-41, 234; GV-13, 75; GV-14, 74; GV-20, 13; GV-4, 78; HT-8, 112; KI-6, 144; KI-8, 146; LI-13, 119; LI-5, 116; LU-11, 102; LU-5, 99; LU-8, 101; LV-13, 48; PC-5, 104; SI-2, 191; SI-4, 126; TW-2, 121; TW-3, 122; TW-4, 122
malaria attack, BL-38, 95
malaria with cold feeling, SI-1, 125
malaria with cold sensations and high fevers, SI-3, 125
malaria with high fever, GV-2, 79

malaria without appetite, ST-44, 152
maries disease, LU-7, 100
mastitis, ST-18, 46
melancholia, BL-14, 238; BL-37, 241; BL-4, 236; BL-41, 242; BL-6, 237; BL-67, 159; GB-12, 228; GB-8, 226; GV-18, 172; LU-10, 176; LU-4, 175; ST-23, 219; ST-36, 150; ST-41, 151; TW-15, 188; GB-6, 225
melancholia and crazed speech, SP-4, 133
melancholia and full feeling in chest, LI-11, 118
melancholia and full feelings in chest with thirst, KI-2, 142
melancholia in chest, HT-7, 111; CV-19, 169; GV-28, 173; KI-1, 141; KI-21, 201; LU-2, 174; SI-1, 125; SP-3, 204; BL-40, 241
melancholia in chest and abdominal pains during menstruation, KI-5, 196
melancholia under the chest area, LU-7, 100; LU-11, 102; KI-19, 200
meningitis, GV-4, 78; KI-1, 141; LU-11, 102
menorrhagia, BL-55, 245; CV-2, 62; CV-3, 61; CV-7, 57; GV-4, 78; LV-1, 137; LV-2, 137; LV-3, 138; SP-10, 135; ST-30, 68
menorrhagia after childbirth, LV-6, 211
menorrhalgia, See also: dysmenorrhea, menstruation
menorrhalgia, CV-2, 62; BL-31, 91; BL-32, 91; BL-33, 92; BL-34, 92; HT-5, 109; KI-14, 198; SP-2, 132; SP-6, 134; ST-44, 152; XT-1, 153
menorrhalgia with a big clot in the uterus, PC-5, 104
menorrhea, HT-5, 109
menstrual cramps, CV-7, 57; SP-6, 134
menstrual cycle, extensive duration and flow scanty, CV-4, 60; SP-6, 134; LV-1, 137; LV-2, 137
menstruation excessive, SP-1, 132
menstruation irregular, CV-3, 61; CV-4, 60; CV-6, 58; GB-26, 49; GB-41, 234; KI-12, 198; KI-13, 198; KI-14, 198; KI-15, 199; KI-5, 196; KI-6, 144; KI-7, 145; LV-5, 211; LV-9, 212; ST-25, 66; ST-28, 67
metritis, BL-30, 90; BL-31, 91; BL-32, 91; BL-33, 92; BL-34, 92; HT-7, 111; PC-5, 104; SP-10, 135
micturition, See also: urination, retention
migraine, See also: headache
migraine, GB-20, 19; GB-4, 224; GB-6, 225; GV-19, 13; LI-4, 115; LU-7, 100; XF-2, 37
migraine headache associated with the neck, GB-17, 228
migraine headache causing the outer canthus to be red/painful, GB-5, 225
miscarriage, CV-8, 55
moral depression, HT-1, 177
morning sickness, PC-5, 104; XT-1, 153

Mouth

mouth abscess, PC-8, 106
mouth and face problem, every kind, LI-4, 115
mouth and lips dry, LI-3, 179
mouth and tongue dry, BL-13, 83
mouth cannot open, LI-4, 115
mouth dry, GB-44, 165; ST-19, 217; LI-1, 115; PC-7, 105; SI-1, 125; TW-4, 122; KI-8, 146; LI-2, 179
mouth dry and very thirsty, LV-14, 46
small ulcers at the outer corners of the mouth, TW-1, 121
mouth paralyzed, LI-19, 184
moving pains, BL-67, 159
moving sensation in the head, XH-2, 35

Moxa Contraindicated

moxa contraindicated, BL-1, 26; BL-2, 25; GB-1, 27; GB-33, 162; GV-15, 18; GV-23, 11; GV-25, 29; GV-28, 173; LI-20, 29; LU-11, 102; LU-5, 99; LU-8, 101; PC-9, 107; TW-23, 26; XF-4, 38; XF-5, 38; XF-6, 38; XF-7, 39; XFi-4, 129; XP-1, 64;
moxa contraindicated during pregnancy, CV-11, 53; CV-4, 60
moxa contraindicated in young males, GV-4, 78
moxa contraindicated, limited use only, LI-15, 72
moxa contraindicated, loss of speech, GV-16, 17
moxa contraindicated, may cause blindness, ST-8, 16
moxa contraindicated, pregnancy and after, SP-2, 132
moxa contraindicated, wet dreams, CV-4, 60
moxa contraindicated, will cause blindness, GB-15, 14

moxa contraindicated, will cause death, GV-26, 31
moxa contraindicated, women, CV-5, 59
mucus (thick) from the nose, GB-5, 225
mucus in the throat causing coughing, LI-3, 179
mumps, TW-17, 22
muscle pain and neuralgia of the shoulder/arm, SI-14, 194
muscle-like vasculature growing from canthus to iris pterygium, BL-1, 26
muscles in shin area withering, ST-40, 151
muscles twitching, BL-65, 249
muscular spasms in general, BL-53, 245
muteness, GV-16, 17; LI-4, 115; TW-6, 123; TW-8, 185
muteness (sudden), HT-4, 109; HT-5, 109; HT-6, 110; HT-7, 111; KI-1, 141; LI-17, 183; LI-18, 183; ST-40, 151; KI-20, 200
myopia, BL-9, 238; GB-1, 27; GB-14, 25; ST-3, 214
nasal abscess, BL-4, 236
nasal catarrh, LI-19, 184
nasal occlusion, GV-20, 13
nasal polyps, GV-23, 11; GV-28, 173; LI-19, 184; LI-20, 29
nausea, HT-1, 177; LU-4, 175

Neck

See also: pain, inflammation, swelling
neck and chest swollen with full feelings in the chest, ST-45, 153
neck sores, SI-7, 192
neck stiff, BL-37, 241; BL-65, 249; GB-13, 16; GB-39, 164; SI-16, 194; SI-7, 192; BL-64, 248; BL-66, 249; GV-18, 172; TW-15, 188
neck stiff cannot turn, GB-19, 229; TW-16, 188
neck tumors, TW-13, 187
neck weakness of or lack of energy in, GB-20, 19

Needle Contraindicated

needle contraindicated, BL-56, 246; BL-6, 237; CV-15, 51; CV-17, 43; CV-8, 55; GB-18, 228; GV-11, 76; GV-17, 172; HT-2, 177; KI-11, 197; LI-4, 115; LU-2, 174; LV-12, 212; ST-1, 213; ST-2, 213; TW-16, 188; TW-7, 185; TW-8, 185; XA-2, 127; XB-1, 96; XFi-2, 128; XFi-3, 128; XFi-5, 130; XH-1, 34; XL-2, 149; XL-3, 157; XSC-1, 63; XT-1, 153
needle contraindicated at evening, GV-24, 11
needle contraindicated during pregnancy, CV-4, 60; ST-25, 66; BL-60, 158; GB-21, 71; SP-6, 134
needle contraindicated more than twice, PC-8, 106
needle contraindicated with heart problems, GB-21, 71
needle contraindicated with nasal polyps, PC-8, 106
needle contraindicated, women, CV-5, 59
nerve weakness of the entire body, GV-20, 13

Neuralgia

See also: pain
neuralgia and paralysis of the face, ST-4, 31
neuralgia of the face, HT-3, 108
neuralgia or cramp in sacrum, BL-30, 90
neuralgia/numbness of the shoulder/arm, SI-13, 193
supraorbital neuralgia, BL-2, 25
neurasthenia, BL-38, 95; GV-11, 76; GV-12, 76; SP-2, 132; ST-36, 150
neuritis or inflammation of the knees, GV-3, 79
night sweating, BL-17, 84; BL-38, 95; KI-7, 145; KI-8, 146; BL-54, 155; SI-3, 125; HT-6, 110; KI-2, 142
night urine, BL-23, 88
nightmares, BL-2, 25
no perspiration, ST-39, 222
no perspiration following the flu, ST-36, 150
noise in the throat, CV-22, 42
noises from breathing, PC-1, 178
nose bleed, BL-12, 83; GB-20, 19; GV-14, 74; GV-15, 18; GV-16, 17; GV-20, 13
nose blocked, BL-3, 236; GB-15, 14; GB-20, 19; GV-16, 17; GV-25, 29; GV-28, 173; KI-22, 201; LI-19, 184; XF-3, 37
nose bulbous from excessive drinking, GV-25, 29
nose catarrh, LI-20, 29
nose problems, BL-12, 83; XF-5, 38
nose stuffed/bleeding, GB-18, 228
nose stuffed, BL-4, 236; BL-6, 237; BL-67, 159; BL-7, 237; GV-25, 29; HT-7, 111; KI-24, 202; LI-20, 29; LI-4, 115; XH-3, 35

nose stuffed and anosmia, BL-9, 238
nose stuffed (tears), BL-10, 18
nose runny, BL-12, 83; BL-6, 237; GB-20, 19; GV-21, 12; GV-25, 29; TW-22, 190
nostrils dry, GB-39, 164

Numbness

numbness, LI-8, 181
numbness below lumbar area, GV-2, 79
numbness from the elbow crease to the hand, PC-3, 103
numbness from the waist down, BL-32, 91
numbness in back and leg, ST-37, 221
numbness in the four limbs, LI-9, 181
numbness in the hip joint, BL-52, 245
numbness in the leg, BL-53, 245; ST-38, 222
numbness in the throat, BL-54, 155; SI-1, 125; ST-36, 150; ST-40, 151; ST-45, 153; TW-1, 121; LI-11, 118; LI-4, 115; LU-5, 99; LU-7, 100; PC-7, 105; ST-39, 222
numbness of arm, LI-10, 117
numbness of face, CV-24, 32; ST-8, 16
numbness of knee/leg with difficulty walking, SP-7, 204
numbness of the bladder where the patient cannot urinate, CV-6, 58
numbness of the chest, LU-9, 101
numbness of the four limbs, BL-30, 90
numbness of the heart, BL-13, 83; BL-17, 84
numbness of the knee, LV-7, 139
numbness of the leg, GB-31, 162; GB-33, 162
numbness of the thigh and knee with cold sensations, ST-31, 220
numbness of vagina, KI-1, 141
numbness with the feeling of insects crawling under the skin, LI-20, 29
nystagmus, ST-4, 31
optic atrophy, GB-1, 27; TW-23, 26
organs congealed and swollen, BL-22, 87
outer canthus, GB-6, 225
outer canthus painful, GB-44, 165
outer canthus red, GB-43, 235
outer corners of eye red and swollen, GB-1, 27; TW-10, 186
ovaritis, ST-27, 67; XT-1, 153
overcooling or overheating, KI-3, 143
overcooling, GB-8, 226; GV-10, 77; SP-21, 210; XF-2, 37

Pain

Pain, See also: neuralgia, lumbago, sore, swelling and the indvidual entries for each anatomical area: arm, back, chest, elbow, eyes, hand, legs, neck, etc. *The following entries relative to pain are grouped in anatomical areas.*

Pain: abdomen, groin area.

pain and coldness around umbilicus, CV-7, 57
pain and swelling in abdomen, ST-33, 148
pain around the umbilicus, BL-25, 89. CV-9, 54
pain between anus and sexual organ, CV-1, 62
pain in abdomen, KI-8, 146; SP-12, 206; BL-16, 239; CV-10, 54; KI-17, 199; SP-13, 206
pain (sharp) in the abdomen like a knife twisting, LI-8, 181
pain in abdomen, groin, umbilical region, KI-3, 143; ST-45, 153; LI-8, 181; BL-23, 88; ST-37, 221
pain in diaphragm, SP-17, 208
pain in genitals, LV-3, 138
pain in intestines, GV-4, 78; BL-27, 89; ST-37, 221
pain in lower abdomen, GB-26, 49; BL-25, 89; KI-7, 145; ST-25, 66; BL-28, 90; KI-6, 144; SI-8, 127; SP-4, 133; GB-25, 231; LV-1, 137; LV-6, 211; LV-8, 139;
pain in the lower abdomen (violent), LV-5, 211
pain in lower abdomen radiating to the throat, ST-31, 220
pain in lower abdomen felt up to the chest, KI-18, 200
lines of pain around the navel, CV-4, 60
loin pain, BL-29, 240; BL-47, 97
loins and back painful, GV-9, 77; GB-27, 231
loins and back stiff/painful, GV-5, 171
loins and chest painful, PC-7, 105
loins and legs painful, GB-32, 232
pain in penis, KI-12, 198; LU-7, 100; LV-1, 137; LV-8, 139; SP-6, 134; ST-29, 68; ST-30, 68
pain of penis or scrotum, LV-12, 212
pain in sex organs,, BL-23, 88; BL-47, 97
pain in sides radiating to chest, SP-13, 206
pain in small intestine, ST-30, 68

pain in testicles, CV-7, 57; LV-5, 211
pain or inflammation in testicles, ST-27, 67
pain in the upper abdomen, ST-26, 219
pain in the whole belly like a knife turning, CV-7, 57
pain in uterus, GB-26, 49; KI-3, 143; ST-33, 148
pain in vagina, CV-3, 61; ST-29, 68; LV-1, 137
pain in one side of the vagina, BL-55, 245
pain or swelling in vagina, CV-1, 62
pain radiating to the umbilicus, ST-26, 219
pain under umbilicus, SP-6, 134

Pain: arm, hand, shoulders and fingers

pain in inner side of arm, HT-9, 113; PC-2, 178
pain and arthritis on the knuckles, XFi-3, 128
pain and weakness in shoulder and arm, LI-15, 72
pain and/or numbness of arms (cannot elevate), SI-9, 192
pain and soreness of the shoulder, TW-15, 188
pain and swelling under the armpit, BL-53, 245
pain as if the arm were broken, SI-6, 191
pain in arms, SI-1, 125; LU-10, 176; PC-1, 178
pain in arm and/or shoulder, SI-14, 186
elbow pain, HT-9, 113
elbow pain/numbness, LI-12, 182
pain in arm and elbow, HT-5, 109; TW-3, 122; LI-13, 119; TW-1, 121; TW-10, 186
pain in armpit and elbow, SI-8, 127
pain in arm joints, GB-4, 224
pain in elbow, LI-11, 118; ST-41, 151
pain in the elbow the patient cannot bend, PC-3, 103
pain in five fingers, LU-11, 102; XFi-5, 130
pain in five fingers and weakness in hand, TW-5, 123; SI-7, 192
pain in the shoulder, LI-11, 118; BL-37, 241
pain in shoulder and arm, TW-4, 122; TW-14, 187; LI-2, 179; BL-40, 241; GB-21, 71; LU-5, 99
pain in shoulder and elbow, SI-8, 127; LI-6, 180
pain in lateral side of the arms, LU-9, 101
pain in outer side of the elbow, SI-11, 193
pain in outer wrist, SI-4, 126
pain in outside edge of arm, SI-5, 126
pain in palm, LU-10, 176
pain in wrist joint, LU-9, 101
pain in the upper arm, LI-11, 118
pain in the yin side of the arm, PC-6, 105
pain under the armpit, GB-42, 235

Pain: back, spine

See also: lumbago, sciatica
pain along vertebral column, GV-26, 31; BL-29, 240
pain from base of spine radiating to lower abdomen, LV-9, 212
pain from the lumbar area reaching the lower abdomen, LV-3, 138
pain in back, BL-21, 86; BL-45, 243; BL-50, 155
pain in back and loins, BL-51, 244
pain in back and spine, KI-4, 145; BL-54, 155
pain in back with chills, BL-41, 242
pain in lower back, BL-31, 91; BL-32, 91; BL-33, 92; GV-7, 171
lower limbs painful and/or numb, SP-6, 134
low back pain radiating to the testicles, BL-34, 92
pain in shoulder and back, LU-9, 101; LI-10, 117; LU-1, 47; LU-2, 174
pain in shoulder radiating to the back, ST-19, 217
pain in spine and sacrum, BL-27, 89
pain in spine, GV-12, 76; LU-5, 99; BL-60, 158
pain or cramp in lumbar vertebrae, CV-9, 54

Pain: chest area

breast pain, PC-1, 178
pain and cold feeling below the xiphoid process, CV-6, 58
pain felt from chest to back, BL-12, 83; PC-2, 178; BL-40, 241; BL-60, 158; CV-22, 42; SP-19, 209; ST-13, 216; BL-42, 242
pain from the chest up to the clavicle, LU-9, 101
pain in area below the sternum, LV-3, 138
pain in chest, CV-19, 169; HT-8, 112; LU-4, 175; TW-10, 186; KI-22, 201; LI-9, 181; KI-21, 201

stabbing pain in the chest, ST-40, 151
pain in chest with chills, GB-41, 234
pain in chest and ribs, GB-44, 165; LV-2, 137; HT-1, 177
pain in chest and sides, GB-38, 163; CV-21, 170; KI-19, 200
pain in chest spreading to the sides, TW-19, 189
pain in chest and stomach, SP-3, 204
pain in chest in different areas at different times, GB-43, 235
pain in heart, LV-14, 46; XT-1, 153
pain in heart area, LV-13, 48
pain in ribs, BL-40, 241
pain in sternum, BL-18, 85
pain in stomach, CV-13, 52
pain spreading to the scapula region, TW-13, 187
pain under the chest (severe), BL-46, 243
pain under the chest with low blood pressure, SP-3, 204
local intercostal neuralgia, ST-12, 45

Pain: face, head and neck, shoulder

See also: headache
pain and tightness in the outer canthus, GB-4, 224
pain behind the ear, GB-12, 228
eye pain, GB-11, 227; BL-40, 241; LI-3, 179; BL-67, 159; GB-44, 165; TW-16, 188 ST-5, 214; GB-14, 25; ST-8, 16; HT-5, 109
eye pain (severe), BL-9, 238
eye dizziness with severe pain, BL-60, 158
pain in eyebrow, BL-2, 25
pain in forehead, BL-2, 25
pain in inner ear, TW-21, 21
neck pain, GB-12, 228; GB-36, 233; BL-36, 240
neck pain with chills, TW-10, 186
neck stiff/painful, ST-11, 216
pain in neck, LU-7, 100
pain in neck and back, BL-10, 18
pain in neck and lower jaw, SI-8, 127
pain in neck with chills and fever, ST-5, 214
nose pain, GB-19, 229
pain in throat, LV-7, 139
trigeminal neuralgia, GB-1, 27; SI-18, 195; ST-6, 23; XF-1, 36
pain in scalp, ST-44, 152
pain in the base of the skull, GB-41, 234
pain in the neck and shoulder, SI-16, 194
pain in the top of the head, GB-8, 226
pain in one side of head and neck, GB-4, 224; GB-11, 227
pain in shoulder, GB-29, 232
pain in shoulder, swollen, TW-13, 187
pain in shoulder and ribs, ST-19, 217

Pain: legs, thigh, feet, knee

pain and cold sensations on knees, BL-31, 91
pain and soreness in thigh and knee, ST-40, 151
pain from the shin to the foot, ST-45, 153
pain from thigh to ankle, GB-38, 163
pain of the knee and leg lumbago with cold, ST-34, 220
pain in ankle joints, LV-4, 138; KI-2, 142
hip and thigh pain, BL-59, 247
hip joint pain, BL-54, 155; GB-40, 164
hip (upper) pain, GB-26, 49
pain in hip radiating to the lower abdomen, GB-25, 231
pain in bottom of heel, KI-7, 145
pain in heel, KI-1, 141; KI-3, 143; ST-36, 150
pain in inner thigh, LV-8, 139; KI-10, 197; SP-5, 133; KI-7, 145
pain in inner thigh/knee, SP-8, 205
pain in knee, LV-8, 139; ST-35, 221; SP-3, 204; XL-1a, 149
pain (sharp) in the knee, KI-10, 197
pain in knee joint, XL-1, 148
pain in the inner side of the knee, SP-6, 134
pain,leg, XL-4, 161; BL-64, 248; ST-38, 222
lower leg pain, BL-62, 158
leg painful in different areas at different times, GB-41, 234
pain in the five toes, LV-4, 138; KI-1, 141
pain in sole of foot, KI-3, 143
pain of the inner side of the foreleg, LV-7, 139
pain under the heel, KI-8, 146

Pain: specific pains

pain at base of the two ischium bones, BL-35, 93
pain at the end of the sternum, LV-2, 137
pain behind the clavicle, LI-1, 115
pain felt in urethra just before urination, KI-10, 197

pain from tooth decay, ST-42, 152; CV-24, 32
pain in gums, TW-2, 121; SI-8, 127
pain, general,joint, BL-58, 246
painful joints, body heavy, SP-2, 132; SP-3, 204
pain moving over body joints, GB-38, 163
pain of medial malleolus, LV-3, 138
pain of skin of whole body, CV-1, 62
pain of tibia bone, KI-1, 141
pale face, LI-8, 181; ST-39, 222
palpitations, CV-13, 52; CV-15, 51; HT-5, 109; HT-6, 110; HT-7, 111; KI-4, 145
panting, CV-6, 58; LV-13, 48; SP-9, 135; ST-40, 151
panting with a sensation of a full chest, LU-1, 47

Paralysis

paralysis, GB-31, 162; LI-20, 29
paralysis following stroke, BL-54, 155
paralysis of arm and elbow, SI-4, 126
paralysis of face, ST-6, 23; CV-24, 32; GB-1, 27; TW-17, 22
paralysis of legs, BL-31, 91
paralysis of one side, LI-8, 181
paralysis of one side of face, Bells palsy, GB-2, 21; ST-44, 152; ST-1, 213
paralysis of the face by yawning, KI-20, 200
paranoia, BL-66, 249
parched lips, TW-1, 121
Parkinsons disease, HT-3, 108; ST-33, 148
PC-5 combined with LI-4 TW-17 GB-2 GV-20 for muteness, GV-15, 18
PC-5 with KI-7 and LI-4 to revive the pulse, LI-4, 115
PC-5 with LI-4 and KI-8 for cessation of the pulse, KI-8, 146
PC-5 with ST-45 for morning sickness, XT-1, 153
PC-9 combination with LI-11, LI-4 for double tongue, GV-15, 18
penis feels cold and painful, CV-1, 62
penis, weakness of, XSC-1, 63; XP-1, 64
pericarditis, PC-6, 105; SP-4, 133
perineal area, all diseases of, CV-1, 62
periosteitis (periostitis), BL-17, 84
peritonitis, BL-63, 159; CV-13, 52; LV-14, 46
perspiration, PC-1, 178
perspiration, absence of, TW-15, 188
perspiration excessive, BL-17, 84; GB-38, 163; HT-6, 110; KI-2, 142; SP-14, 207; TW-10, 186
pharyngitis, CV-23, 41; ST-11, 216
pharynx swollen, ST-10, 216
phlegm (thick) in the chest, LU-5, 99
phlegm coming from the mouth, SI-1, 125
phlegm coming from the mouth and lockjaw, TW-1, 121
phlegm excessive, ST-40, 151
phlegm in the stomach, GB-8, 226
piles, BL-50, 155; BL-57, 157; CV-1, 62; GB-39, 164; GV-1, 80; KI-8, 146; PC-4, 103; SP-5, 133; XA-1, 104
piles burning, PC-8, 106
pleurisy, BL-11, 82; BL-12, 83; BL-17, 84; BL-19, 85; CV-18, 169; KI-26, 202; KI-8, 146; LU-1, 47; LU-5, 99; LV-13, 48; LV-14, 46; SP-10, 135; SP-4, 133; ST-12, 45; ST-18, 46; ST-40, 151
pleurisy, swelling of the abdomen, panting and insomnia, SP-1, 132
pneumonia, BL-13, 83; LI-13, 119; LU-1, 47
poison, KI-10, 197
poisonous furuncle on the back, BL-65, 249
poisonous snake bites, LI-5, 116
polyps, GV-25, 29
post-partum troubles such as hiccoughs and belching, LV-14, 46
pre and post partum difficulties, GV-20, 13
pregnancy, sudden anuria, KI-1, 141
pregnant, difficulty breathing and pulling down feelings, SP-12, 206
premature ejaculation, GV-3, 79
premature labor or miscarriage with cold limbs, GB-21, 71
pricking technique, 14, 39
prismatic needle, 14, 39; HT-9, 113; LI-1, 115; TW-1, 121
prismatic needle for inflamation of the eyes, BL-2, 25
prolapse of anus, GV-20, 13; XA-1, 104
prolapse of rectum, CV-4, 60; GV-1, 80
prolapse of uterus, BL-31, 91; CV-1, 62; CV-3, 61; CV-4, 60; HT-8, 112; KI-1, 141; KI-2, 142; KI-5, 196; KI-6, 144; KI-7, 145; LV-8, 139
prolapse of the vagina, BL-32, 91
prolapse, rectal, CV-8, 55
prolapse, rectal, in a child, GV-6, 171

pruritis and pain on the skin, BL-13, 83
pruritis vulvae, CV-1, 62; CV-3, 61
pterygium, BL-18, 85
pulmonary congestion, KI-25, 202
pulmonary emphysema, GV-14, 74
pulse at point, BL-1, 26; BL-2, 25; KI-3, 143; LI-4, 115; LI-5, 116; LU-7, 100; LU-8, 101; LU-9, 101; LV-3, 138; PC-3, 103; ST-12, 45; ST-30, 68; ST-42, 152; ST-5, 214; ST-9, 215; TW-21, 21; TW-22, 190; TW-23, 26; XF-2, 37
pulse not palpable, PC-5, 104
pulse, sudden cessation of, KI-8, 146
purulent rhinitis, GV-23, 11
rabies, GB-36, 233
red and white vaginal discharge, GB-27, 231; SP-10, 135
red and/or white vaginal discharge, CV-6, 58; CV-2, 62; GB-26, 49; GV-4, 78
red eyes, ST-41, 151
red face, CV-6, 58; SI-18, 195; ST-41, 151
red face and excessive laughter, HT-7, 111
red or white dysentery, BL-29, 240
regurgitation of milk, BL-21, 86
relaxing tight muscles of the face, ST-4, 31
retained placenta, BL-60, 158; CV-3, 61; CV-4, 60; KI-6, 144; PC-6, 105; SP-4, 133; ST-30, 68; XT-1, 153
retention of urine, BL-48, 244; CV-2, 62; LI-6, 180; ST-25, 66
retention of urine and feces, ST-28, 67
retinal hemorrhage, GB-1, 27
retinitis, BL-1, 26
retraction of testicle, LV-3, 138
rhinorrhea, LI-20, 29
ringing in the ear, GB-2, 21; SI-4, 126; TW-21, 21
ringworm, TW-6, 123
ringworm itching, PC-7, 105
ringworm on the face of children, GV-28, 173
running around madly, GV-8, 172; LI-8, 181; BL-8, 238
sacral vertebrae, 3
sad always, SP-15, 207
sadness in heart and mind, SP-5, 133
saliva, (clear) dribbling from mouth, LI-8, 181
saliva/spitting, excessive, KI-26, 202
scabies, LI-11, 118; PC-7, 105; SI-3, 125; TW-6, 123

Sciatica

sciatica, BL-30, 90; BL-31, 91; BL-32, 91; BL-33, 92; BL-60, 158; GB-30, 161; GB-32, 232; GB-34, 163; XL-4, 161
scolding, KI-9, 196
scoliosis, XSP-1, 166
scrofula, GV-9, 77; LI-10, 117; LI-11, 118; LI-13, 119; LI-14, 119; LI-15, 72; LU-7, 100; ST-12, 45; ST-5, 214; TW-17, 22; XA-2, 127; XN-1, 34
scrofula on neck, ST-9, 215
scrofula or neck tumor preventing speech, GB-10, 227
scrotum, loosening of scrotum, XSC-1, 63
seasickness and carsickness, PC-5, 104
secretions (excessive female) during intercourse, GB-41, 234; KI-6, 144; KI-7, 145; SP-12, 206; ST-20, 218; GB-37, 234
seeing ghosts, ST-40, 151
sees devils, LI-7, 180
semen comes out cold, BL-23, 88
semen, loss of semen, KI-11, 197
semen runs out uncontrollably, CV-8, 55
sensations in the tibia, LV-6, 211
sexual frigidity, XSC-1, 63
sexual intercourse (the man can not control), CV-8, 55
shakes while standing and cannot stand for a long time, BL-58, 246
shaking, BL-63, 159
shaking of the arm and elbow, PC-3, 103
shaking of the body, BL-57, 157
shaking of the eyeball, ST-1, 213
shaking of the hand, HT-3, 108
shin pain, GB-39, 164; ST-36, 150
shins sore, BL-62, 158; BL-63, 159; KI-2, 142; GB-38, 163
shivering without cold, KI-14, 198
shock, BL-42, 242; BL-61, 247; BL-63, 159; BL-7, 237; LI-19, 184
short-sightedness, GV-23, 11 shortness of breath walking up the stairs, CV-14, 52

Shoulder

See also: pain, swelling, inflammation
shoulder and arm neuralgia and numbness, SI-12, 193
shoulder and elbow numb, BL-36, 240
shoulder and neck stiffness, LI-1, 115
shoulder, spine and loins cannot bend, BL-22, 87

shoulder cramp radiating to the back, BL-36, 240
shoulder hot, SI-13, 193
shoulder numbness/pain on the shoulder, GB-25, 231
shoulders moving up and down during breathing, ST-20, 218
SI-19 used for deafness, treatment note, TW-17, 22
sighing, GB-24, 230; HT-8, 112; LV-2, 137; SP-5, 133
sinking pulse, KI-3, 143
sinusitis, BL-2, 25; GV-24, 11

Skin

skin and flesh painful, TW-7, 185
skin disease/abscess/carbuncle (any), BL-54, 155
skin diseases, BL-17, 84; LI-11, 118; SP-10, 135
skin dropping off, with abscesses, LI-11, 118
skin dry on the legs, GB-42, 235
skin dry with no perspiration, GV-4, 78; BL-19, 85
skin, dryness of, LI-11, 118; BL-38, 95
skin is hard as stone, LV-13, 48
skin painful, GB-36, 233
skin swollen, GB-8, 226
skin tumor on the neck, ST-11, 216
slackness of jaw, GB-2, 21; GV-11, 76; ST-6, 23; TW-17, 22
sleeping, excessive, GV-22, 12; KI-1, 141; KI-6, 144; LI-12, 182; LI-13, 119; LV-10, 212; ST-45, 153; TW-10, 186; TW-8, 185
sleeping patient with little interest in anything except sleeping, KI-3, 143
smell, loss of the sense of, GV-22, 12
smoking, CV-20, 170
sneezing, BL-12, 83; LU-5, 99
sneezing, excessive, GB-4, 224

Sore

See also: pain
sore and painful foot, KI-3, 143
soreness/numbness of the foot, ST-44, 152
sore and painful on tibia bone, LV-3, 138; ST-37, 221
sore and painful shoulder and upper arm, SI-6, 191
sore arms, HT-8, 112
sore shins, BL-57, 157
sore throat, LU-6, 175
sores, GV-28, 173
sorrowful, GB-39, 164; ST-15, 217
sound in the throat during breathing, KI-4, 145
sound during breathing, LI-20, 29; LI-18, 183
sound of water moving around the diaphragm area, SP-17, 208
spasm, SI-14, 194
spasm in the lower abdomen, CV-11, 53
spasm in the vagina, KI-6, 144
spasm of esophagus, LI-2, 179; LU-8, 101
spasm of the legs, SP-3, 204
special point for any disease of the five solid organs, LV-13, 48
special point for double tongue, GV-15, 18
speech difficult, GB-23, 230; GB-24, 230; ST-1, 213; TW-10, 186
spermatorrhea, BL-23, 88; BL-38, 95; BL-47, 97; BL-67, 159; CV-2, 62; CV-3, 61; CV-4, 60; CV-6, 58; GV-4, 78; KI-12, 198; LV-4, 138; LV-8, 139; SP-6, 134
spermatorrhea after talking a long time, LI-15, 72
spermatorrhea caused by fright, GV-1, 80
spine stiff, BL-25, 89; BL-29, 240
spine stiffness, pain or numbness, XSP-1, 166
spirit and chi insufficient, PC-4, 103
spirit, weakness in, GV-24, 11
spirit worried, TW-10, 186
spitting, SP-20, 210
spitting, excessive, BL-41, 242; GB-23, 230; GB-24, 230
spitting, frequent, KI-18, 200; KI-21, 201; SI-1, 125
spitting up pus, TW-10, 186
spitting with blood, KI-3, 143; ST-36, 150
spleen and stomach, weakness of, SP-6, 134
spleen weakness and patient unhappy, SP-5, 133
spotting between periods, KI-10, 197
sputum (thick) with blood/pus, ST-14, 217
sputum with thick phlegm/pus, ST-20, 218
ST-33 and HT-3 for Parkinsons disease, ST-33, 148
ST-36 treatment for weakness, BL-38, 95
ST-44 (one of the eight winds), XFo-1, 165

ST-45 with PC-5 for morning sickness, XT-1, 153
stenosis of the esophagus, BL-15, 84; BL-17, 84; BL-19, 85; CV-16, 43; CV-17, 43; CV-22, 42; KI-4, 145; LU-9, 101; PC-6, 105
sterility, LV-11, 69; ST-25, 66; ST-29, 68; ST-30, 68
sterility in females, BL-31, 91; BL-32, 91; BL-33, 92; KI-1, 141
sterility in males, SP-8, 205
sternum, LV-2, 137

Stiffness

stiffness, GV-2, 79; SI-5, 126
stiff and painful finger joints, XFi-6, 130
stiff arm (as if someone was pulling the arm out), SI-6, 191
stiffness of back, BL-47, 97; BL-41, 242; BL-56, 246
stiffness of five fingers, XFi-5, 130
stiffness of the head and neck, GV-19, 13
stiff lips, GV-27, 173
stiff tongue, CV-22, 42; SI-1, 125
stiffness and/or pain of knuckles, XHn-1, 129
stiffness behind the knee, BL-65, 249
stiffness of shoulder, SI-8, 127
stiffness of the lower back, GV-8, 172
stiffness of the neck, BL-10, 18; BL-7, 237; GB-11, 227; GB-20, 19; GV-16, 17; HT-3, 108; SI-3, 125; ST-6, 23; XN-1, 34; GV-15, 18; GB-7, 226; SI-1, 125
stiffness of neck and back, BL-13, 83
stiffness of the neck after the flu, BL-12, 83
stiffness of the neck and coughing, BL-11, 82
stiffness of the shoulder and back, BL-60, 158
stiffness of the spine, KI-18, 200; LI-4, 115
stiffness of the upper lip, GB-3, 224
stiffness of upper thigh, ST-31, 220
stiffness on back and spine with pain, BL-55, 245
stiffness on the chest or back, LU-8, 101
stiffness or cramping of neck, LI-14, 119; GB-21, 71

Stomach

stomach cancer, SP-4, 133
stomach cramps, GV-6, 171
stomach diseases, CV-12, 53; PC-6, 105
stomach distended (woman) touching it creates a wave, SP-8, 205
stomach enlarged, SP-10, 135
stomach feels cold, cannot eat, GV-9, 77
stomach feels full and hot with pain, CV-7, 57
stomach or intestines, any disease of, CV-8, 55
stomach, overfull feeling in, LU-11, 102
stomach pains with anorexia, LU-10, 176
stomach problems, acute or chronic, ST-25, 66
stomach swollen as in pregnancy but from worms, KI-10, 197
stomach swollen similar to dropsy, KI-10, 197
stomach, weakness of the, BL-20, 86
stomachache, BL-21, 86; CV-10, 54; GV-7, 171; SP-4, 133; ST-44, 152
stools, See also: diarrhea
stools contain undigested food, BL-20, 86; BL-23, 88; BL-25, 89
stools green (children), BL-21, 86

Stroke

See also: apoplexy, hemiplegia
stroke, XFi-4, 129
stroke, beginning of stroke unconscious patient with phlegm, PC-9, 107; PC-5, 104; HT-9, 113
stroke, difficulty breathing wih phlegm in the mouth GB-21, 71; GB-20, 19
stroke, beginning of a stroke, LU-11, 102; SI-1, 125; TW-1, 121
stroke, mouth closed, ST-5, 214; LI-1, 115
stroke patient crying and laughing or talking nonsense LU-3, 174,
stroke, arm is paralyzed, LI-10, 117
stroke, patient is very angry, PC-8, 106
sunstroke, GB-20, 19; XFi-4, 129
sweating and pruritis of the scrotum, CV-7, 57
sweating, excessive, KI-8, 146; SI-3, 125
sweating from genitals, BL-35, 93

Swelling

swelling and pain in arms, ST-18, 46
swelling in abdomen, CV-8, 55; KI-8, 146; ST-30, 68; LV-1, 137; SP-3, 204; ST-44, 152
lower abdomen swollen or full and extremely painful, CV-2, 62

swelling in lower abdomen, ST-27, 67; LV-8, 139; KI-2, 142; LV-3, 138; KI-11, 197; LV-2, 137; LV-4, 138
swelling in lower abdomen (women), ST-28, 67
swelling in the abdomen and loins, LV-8, 139
swelling in the abdomen with gas, LV-13, 48
swelling in the abdomen with sounds in the intestines, LV-13, 48
swelling in the abdomen causing back pain, BL-20, 86
swollen abdomen with lumbago, KI-1, 141
swelling under the armpits, BL-19, 85; PC-5, 104; PC-1, 178; PC-7, 105; BL-56, 246; GB-38, 163; GB-40, 164
swelling of ankle joints, KI-2, 142
body swollen, ST-22, 218
swelling of breasts, ST-36, 150; SP-18, 209
swelling of buttocks, BL-50, 155; BL-49, 244
swelling of chest and abdomen, GB-39, 164
chest under sternum hard and swollen, BL-32, 91
swelling under the chest, LU-11, 102
swelling of elbow, PC-5, 104
swollen face with feeling of insects crawling in skin, GV-26, 31
swelling of face, LI-20, 29; LI-4, 115; CV-24, 32; ST-41, 151; ST-45, 153; XF-6, 38
swelling on face and arms, LU-1, 47
swelling of the face and eyes, GV-21, 12
swelling of head and face, GB-16, 14; GB-12, 228; GB-34, 163
swelling top of head, BL-4, 236
swelling of four limbs, LU-1, 47; ST-40, 151
swelling of the four limbs (sudden maries' disease), LU-7, 100
swelling in the throat, GV-15, 18; KI-3, 143; TW-3, 122
swelling, numb throat, CV-20, 170
swelling of throat with dyspnea, KI-1, 141
swelling in the tongue, LU-11, 102; LI-7, 180
swelling of jaw, ST-6, 23; LI-1, 115; LI-10, 117; LI-2, 179; ST-4, 31; GB-7, 226
swelling of jaw with pain radiating behind the ear, SI-2, 191
swelling of knee (crane knee), XL-1, 148; ST-35, 221
sweling of larynx, ST-9, 215
swelling of legs, LV-3, 138
swelling of lips, LI-20, 29
swelling of loins, SP-9, 135
neck swollen and painful, SI-10, 192; TW-12, 187
swelling of neck, SI-4, 126; SI-5, 126; SI-8, 127; GB-40, 164; SI-2, 191; TW-22, 190
swelling of the ribs, ST-16, 45; GB-41, 234
swelling of the skin on head, GV-22, 12
swelling of the spleen, LV-13, 48
swollen upper abdomen and sides, LV-3, 138
swelling of the upper abdomen, CV-14, 52; ST-36, 150
swelling and soreness, BL-55, 245
swollen scrotum, LV-1, 137
swollen scrotum with fluid, SP-10, 135
swollen sex organs, BL-47, 97; LV-8, 139
swollen and painful vaginal orifice, CV-3, 61
syphilitic buboes, BL-57, 157
talking with cardiac pain, GV-8, 172
tapeworm, ST-25, 66
taste, loss of taste, ST-13, 216
tearing, excessive, LV-2, 137
tearing with dizziness, BL-2, 25
tears excessive, GB-15, 14; GB-20, 19; ST-8, 16
tears flow in bright light, TW-23, 26
tears flow in wind, BL-1, 26
terror, TW-18, 189
testicle and scrotum (any problem of), XSC-1, 63
testicle retracts into the body from cramping, CV-6, 58
testicles retract into the body, ST-30, 68; LV-4, 138; GB-27, 231; ST-29, 68
testicles, inflammation of, XL-3, 157
tetanus in children, KI-2, 142
thigh and knee, weakness of, GB-31, 162
thigh and leg numb, BL-56, 246
thigh cramps, ST-41, 151
thigh numb, GB-34, 163
thigh sore, BL-56, 246
thighs swollen, BL-51, 244
thinking, excessive, SP-5, 133

thirst, BL-23, 88; BL-29, 240; BL-44, 243; CV-24, 32; LU-11, 102; SI-7, 192; TW-4, 122
thirst (severe), BL-27, 89
thirst and frequent, difficult urination, ST-27, 67
thirst excessive, GV-26, 31; GV-27, 173; XF-7, 39
thirst, but cannot eat or drink, PC-8, 106
thoracic vertebrae, 3

Throat

throat and jaw swollen, LU-11, 102
throat and mouth dryness, LV-3, 138; HT-9, 113; LU-9, 101; KI-6, 144; LU-10, 176
throat, closing of, TW-1, 121
throat dry and numb, LI-6, 180
throat sensation of something caught in the throat, PC-5, 104; SI-17, 195; LI-3, 179
throat inflamed, GB-11, 227
throat numb, GB-35, 233; GB-38, 163; GB-39, 164; GB-44, 165; LI-2, 179; LI-7, 180; LV-3, 138; SI-17, 195; SI-2, 191
throat numb and swollen, TW-10, 186; CV-21, 170; ST-11, 216
throat, numb swollen throat with dyspnea, LI-17, 183
throat problems, BL-54, 155
throat swollen, CV-22, 42; ST-11, 216
throat swollen and fluid does not descend, CV-15, 51
throat swollen and painful, GV-16, 17
tibia area, BL-55, 245; ST-38, 222
tibia sore, GB-41, 234
tight sensation in the chest during the flu, TW-6, 123
tinnitus, BL-8, 238; GB-10, 227; GB-20, 19; GB-3, 224; GB-4, 224; GV-4, 78; LI-1, 115; LI-5, 116; SI-17, 195; SI-19, 22; SI-2, 191; SI-5, 126; SI-9, 192; ST-1, 213; TW-17, 22; TW-18, 189; TW-19, 189; TW-22, 190
tinnitus causing deafness, GB-10, 227; GB-11, 227
tired, BL-17, 84
tongue, CV-23, 41; SI-5, 126
tongue cannot retract into mouth, SI-5, 126; LI-3, 179
tongue curled up, TW-1, 121
tongue dry, BL-19, 85; GV-27, 173; KI-4, 145
tongue, erosion on the surface of, TW-1, 121
tongue hanging out and patient dribbling saliva, KI-10, 197
tongue loose, CV-23, 41
tongue moves slowly, GV-15, 18
tongue stiff, CV-23, 41; GB-44, 165; KI-1, 141; ST-24, 219; ST-5, 214
tongue stiff and painful, SP-5, 133
tongue stretched out, KI-9, 196; ST-23, 219; ST-24, 219
tongue swollen, PC-9, 107
tongue swollen and painful, 14, 39
tonsillitis, BL-19, 85; CV-16, 43; CV-20, 170; CV-21, 170; GB-10, 227; HT-5, 109; HT-6, 110; HT-7, 111; KI-1, 141; KI-2, 142; KI-6, 144; LI-1, 115; LI-2, 179; LI-3, 179; LI-4, 115; LI-6, 180; LI-7, 180; LU-1, 47; LU-2, 174; LU-6, 175; LU-8, 101; SI-16, 194; ST-44, 152; XFi-4, 129
tooth decay, GB-3, 224
toothache, BL-14, 238; CV-24, 32; GB-10, 227; GB-12, 228; GB-17, 228; GV-16, 17; LI-1, 115; LI-10, 117; LI-2, 179; LI-3, 179; LI-4, 115; LI-6, 180; SI-5, 126; ST-4, 31; ST-44, 152; ST-45, 153; XHn-1, 129
toothache of lower jaw, LI-16, 72; ST-6, 23; TW-9, 185
toothache of upper jaw, GV-26, 31; TW-21, 21
torticollis, BL-10, 18
trigeminal neuralgia, GB-1, 27; SI-18, 195; ST-6, 23; XF-1, 36
tuberculosis, BL-12, 83; BL-13, 83; BL-15, 84; BL-23, 88; BL-38, 95; GB-19, 229; GV-12, 76; GV-13, 75; GV-14, 74; KI-1, 141; LI-10, 117; LU-1, 47; LU-5, 99; LU-7, 100; XB-2, 97
tuberculosis with diarrhea, LI-8, 181

Tumor

See also: cancer
tumor, fatty on skin, LI-15, 72; BL-13, 83
tumor in abdomen, CV-10, 54
tumor on the skin, LU-1, 47
soft tumor under the tongue, LU-11, 102
small neck tumor, SI-7, 192
tumors, any, XB-1, 96
TW-17 combined with PC-5, LI-4, GB-2, GV-20 for muteness, GV-15, 18

TW-17 used for deafness (treatment note), TW-17, 22
TW-2, TW-3 used with XH-1, XHn-1, 129
TW-21 used for deafness (treatment note), TW-17, 22
TW-5 in combination with LU-11 for weakness of hand, TW-5, 123
twisting of face, GB-13, 16
twisting or spasm of one side of the face, XH-2, 35
typhoid fever, XFi-4, 129
uncomfortable feeling in chest, TW-4, 122; TW-6, 123
uncomfortable feelings in the heart, LU-5, 99
unconscious, SP-1, 132; SP-6, 134
unconscious from apoplexy, CV-8, 55
unconsciousness from shock, sudden, CV-1, 62
uncontrollable streams of cold tears, SI-4, 126
underdevelopment of the brain in children, GV-20, 13
unhappy and distant from reality, BL-8, 238

Urination

urination, See also: night urine, retention
urinary incontinence, BL-53, 245; CV-3, 61;
CV-4, 60; HT-8, 112
urination and defecation difficult, BL-25, 89; GV-1, 80; ST-40, 151
urination at night, frequency of, CV-4, 60
urination difficult, LI-9, 181
urination difficult with deep yellow or red colored urine, CV-5, 59
urination frequent, CV-3, 61; KI-5, 196; GV-5, 171; LV-1, 137
urination from coughing, LU-10, 176
urination, weak force of, XSC-1, 63
urine, burning sensation while urinating, LU-7, 100
urine cloudy, XH-1, 34
urine deep yellow, ST-45, 153; GV-27, 173; KI-18, 200
urine flow irregular, speed of, BL-33, 92; BL-47, 97
urine icteric or red, BL-28, 90; BL-41, 242; BL-42, 242; LI-9, 181; GB-12, 228; GB-25, 231; BL-44, 243
urticaria, KI-1, 141; LI-4, 115
urticaria of the entire body, GB-30, 161
uterine prolapse, GB-26, 49
uterus does not reduce in size after childbirth, CV-2, 62
uterus pain, BL-62, 158
uterus tipped, LV-11, 69; ST-30, 68
vaginal bleeding, GV-20, 13
vaginal discharge, CV-4, 60; CV-7, 57; KI-12, 198; LV-5, 211
vaginal discharge, white and red, SP-6, 134
vaginal discharge, white or red, BL-23, 88
vaginal odors (special treatment for), HT-9, 113
vertigo, BL-7, 237; GB-13, 16; GB-16, 14; GV-16, 17; GV-18, 172; GV-19, 13; GV-22, 12; XF-3, 37
vertigo and headache, BL-10, 18
visceroptosis, CV-8, 55

Vision

vision poor (night), BL-1, 26; GB-14, 25; LV-2, 137; BL-2, 25; GB-1, 27; GB-20, 19; ST-1, 213; ST-4, 31
vision, night blindness of children, BL-21, 86
vision, stars in, KI-6, 144
vision abnormal, GV-1, 80; LI-2, 179; GB-16, 14; BL-2, 25; PC-1, 178; PC-2, 178
vision dim; BL-1, 26; BL-15, 84; BL-5, 236; BL-66, 249; GB-3, 224; LI-4, 115; LI-6, 180; LU-3, 174; SI-15, 194; SI-6, 191; ST-1, 213; ST-2, 213; TW-16, 188
visited by spectres, LI-5, 116
voice, loss of, KI-1, 141; LU-6, 175

Vomiting

vomiting, BL-12, 83; BL-13, 83; BL-14, 238; BL-17, 84; BL-20, 86; BL-21, 86; BL-22, 87; BL-37, 241; BL-41, 242; BL-44, 243; BL-6, 237; BL-61, 247; CV-10, 54; CV-11, 53; CV-14, 52; CV-16, 43; CV-22, 42; CV-23, 41; CV-6, 58; GB-23, 230; GB-28, 232; GB-8, 226; GV-14, 74; KI-24, 202; KI-25, 202; KI-26, 202; KI-27, 203; KI-3, 143; KI-4, 145; KI-6, 144; LU-8, 101; LV-13, 48; PC-3, 103; SI-17, 195; SP-3, 204; SP-4, 133; SP-5, 133; ST-36, 150; ST-9, 215; TW-18, 189; XF-3, 37
vomiting (unceasing), GB-28, 232
vomiting (severe), ST-24, 219; XFi-2, 128
vomiting alot of mucus, LI-18, 183

vomiting after eating, BL-13, 83; LV-14, 46; PC-5, 104; KI-20, 200
vomiting and anorexia, SP-1, 132
vomiting and body feels cold, LV-3, 138
vomiting and diarrhea in children (severe), SP-1, 132
vomiting blood, CV-13, 52; CV-19, 169; CV-5, 59; GV-1, 80; LI-16, 72; PC-4, 103; ST-19, 217; ST-20, 218
vomiting cold phlegm, CV-18, 169
vomiting, diarrhea and abdominal pain, SP-3, 204
vomiting, dry, BL-19, 85; HT-4, 109; PC-5, 104
vomiting food, CV-19, 169
vomiting mucus, GV-18, 172
vomiting of excessive saliva and mucus with madness, TW-23, 26
vomiting of milk by children, CV-16, 43
vomiting of stomach liquid, SP-6, 134
vomiting of thick phlegm, CV-19, 169
vomiting saliva, KI-9, 196
vomiting saliva in children, TW-19, 189
vomiting sour tasting vomit, LV-14, 46
vomiting with bubbly saliva, LU-7, 100; PC-5, 104
vomiting with phlegm, CV-13, 52; ST-19, 217
vomiting with phlegm and pus, CV-17, 43
vomiting with saliva/phlegm, KI-21, 201
walking difficult, BL-55, 245
walks about madly, ST-23, 219
walks around madly, GV-19, 13
water sound in the intestines, CV-8, 55
water stagnates in the stomach, BL-66, 249; KI-20, 200
weak sense of smell, BL-10, 18
weakness following recovery from a disease, BL-38, 95
weakness in the five viscera, CV-2, 62
weakness of the entire body (severe), CV-4, 60
weakness of the leg, GB-32, 232
weeping excessive, GV-28, 173
wet dreams, BL-15, 84; BL-23, 88; BL-47, 97; BL-38, 95; KI-2, 142; CV-4, 60; SP-6, 134; SP-9, 135
wet dreams with excessive loss of semen, CV-6, 58
wheezing, LI-17, 183
wheezing from bronchi, SP-18, 209
wheezing in the throat, LU-11, 102
whole body swollen, ST-20, 218
whooping cough, BL-12, 83; SP-5, 133
wind causing the eyes to water, GB-20, 19
worms moving in the stomach and excessive saliva, KI-8, 146
worrying in the heart, PC-7, 105
wrist, weakness or pain in the, TW-4, 122
XH-1, TW-3 used with TW-2, XHn-1, 129
yang chi empty, penis is weak, CV-6, 58
yang, losing of the yang, CV-8, 55; GV-1, 80; ST-28, 67
yawning in infants, TW-17, 22
yellow coating of the tongue, LU-10, 176 PC-5, 104; PC-6, 105
yellow/red dysentery, BL-43, 242

Pain Index

lumbar	ache, BL-25, 89; GB-25, 231; XB-2, 97
lower lumbar	ache, BL-31, 91; BL-32, 91; BL-33, 92
	lumbago, BL-24, 239; BL-26, 239; BL-29, 240; BL-49, 244; BL-56, 246; BL-57, 157; BL-59, 247; BL-28, 90; BL-62, 158; BL-64, 248; GB-31, 162; GB-34, 163; GB-38, 163; GB-39, 164; GV-26, 31; GV-3, 79; KI-1, 141; KI-3, 143; LV-2, 137; SP-2, 132; SP-9, 135; ST-31, 220; ST-36, 150; TW-10, 186
swollen abdomen with	lumbago, KI-1, 141
	lumbago reacting to the knee, GB-30, 161
pain of the knee and leg	lumbago with cold, ST-34, 220
kidneys, weakness of with	lumbar ache, BL-23, 88; GV-4, 78
	lumbar ache, BL-25, 89; GB-25, 231; XB-2, 97
lower	lumbar ache, BL-31, 91; BL-32, 91; BL-33, 92
	lumbar and thigh painful, GB-40, 164
heavy feelings in the	lumbar area, BL-54, 155
numbness below	lumbar area, GV-2, 79
sitting in cold water	lumbar area cold and sore as if, GB-38, 163
	lumbar area cold like ice, BL-23, 88
abdomen	pain from the lumbar area reaching the lower, LV-3, 138
	lumbar area stiff, GV-1, 80
	lumbar pain, GV-2, 79
	lumbar, thigh, knees cold like water, ST-33, 148
trigeminal	neuralgia, GB-1, 27; SI-18, 195; ST-6, 23; XF-1, 36
pain or cramp in	lumbar vertebrae, CV-9, 54
cardiac	pain, BL-16, 239; BL-64, 248; CV-14, 52; GV-8, 172;
intercostal	pain, BL-18, 85; HT-2, 177
the abdomen causing back	pain, swelling, BL-20, 86
loin	pain, BL-29, 240; BL-47, 97
gastric	pain, BL-43, 242; CV-15, 51; KI-18, 200; SP-2, 132; ST-43, 223
back	pain, BL-44, 243; GB-20, 19; GV-2, 79; KI-8, 146; SP-8, 205
knee	pain, BL-54, 155; GB-35, 233; GB-37, 234; LV-2, 137; LV-7, 139; ST-38, 222; ST-45, 153
hip joint	pain, BL-54, 155; GB-40, 164
stiff back and spine with	pain, BL-55, 245
heel	pain, BL-56, 246; BL-57, 157; BL-61, 247; ST-39, 222
joint	pain, BL-58, 246
calf	pain, BL-58, 246; KI-9, 196
hip and thigh	pain, BL-59, 247
eye dizziness with severe	pain, BL-60, 158
lower leg	pain, BL-62, 158
uterus	pain, BL-62, 158
forehead	pain, BL-63, 159
stomach full, hot with	pain, CV-7, 57
eye	pain, GB-11, 227; BL-40, 241; LI-3, 179; BL-67, 159; GB-44, 165; TW-16, 188; ST-5, 214; GB-14, 25; ST-8, 16; HT-5, 109
neck	pain, GB-12, 228; GB-36, 233.
nose	pain, GB-19, 229
lower quadrant	pain, GB-26, 49
shoulder	pain, GB-29, 232

shin	pain, GB-39, 164; ST-36, 150
lumbar	pain, GV-2, 79
talking with cardiac	pain, GV-8, 172
elbow	pain, HT-9, 113
back, lower back	pain, KI-12, 198
arm	pain, LI-12, 182; LI-14, 119; SI-2, 191; TW-13, 187
vaginal	pain, LV-1, 137
intestinal	pain, LV-1, 137; LV-2, 137; SP-6, 134; ST-22, 218
local	pain, LV-11, 69; XF-3, 37
breast	pain, PC-1, 178
inner foot	pain, SP-5, 133
full feeling in chest with	pain, ST-18, 46
elbow/arm	pain, TW-10, 186
leg	pain, XL-4, 161; BL-64, 248; ST-38, 222
	pain along the inside of the arm, PC-2, 178
	pain along vertebral column, GV-26, 31; BL-29, 240
knuckles	pain and arthritis on the, XFi-3, 128
xiphoid process	pain and cold feeling below the, CV-6, 58
	pain and cold sensations on knees, BL-31, 91
umbilicus	pain and coldness around, CV-7, 57
shoulder/arm	muscle pain and neuralgia of the, SI-14, 194
intercostal	pain and numbness, ST-18, 46
knee	pain and soreness in thigh and, ST-40, 151
	pain and soreness of the shoulder, TW-15, 188
	pain and swelling in abdomen, ST-33, 148
armpit	pain and swelling under the, BL-53, 245
outer canthus	pain and tightness in, GB-4, 224
arm	pain and weakness in shoulder and, LI-15, 72
(cannot elevate)	pain and/or numbness of arms, SI-9, 192
lines of	pain around the navel, CV-4, 60
umbilicus	pain around the, CV-9, 54; BL-25, 89.
	pain as if the arm were broken, SI-6, 191
back	pain associated with constipation, SP-3, 204
ischium bones	pain at base of, BL-35, 93
	pain at the end of the sternum, LV-2, 137
gas in abdomen causing	pain at the umbilicus, ST-22, 218
	pain behind the clavicle, LI-1, 115
	pain behind the ear, GB-12, 228
sexual organ	pain between anus and, CV-1, 62
cannot open eye	pain, ST-5, 214
cannot turn neck	pain, BL-36, 240
bend, stretch, raise	armpain, LU-6, 175
	pain felt from chest to back, BL-12, 83; PC-2, 178; BL-40, 241; BL-60, 158; CV-22, 42; SP-19, 209; ST-13, 216; BL-42, 242
before urination	pain felt in urethra, KI-10, 197
lower abdomen	pain felt up to the chest, KI-18, 200
to lower abdomen	pain from base of spine radiating, LV-9, 212
clavicle	pain from the chest up to the, LU-9, 101
reaching the lower abdomen	pain from the lumbar area, LV-3, 138
	pain from the shin to the foot, ST-45, 153
	pain from thigh to ankle, GB-38, 163
	pain from tooth decay, ST-42, 152; CV-24, 32

pain in abdomen, KI-8, 146; SP-12, 206; BL-16, 239; CV-10, 54; KI-17, 199; SP-13, 206
pain in abdomen and loins, KI-3, 143
pain in abdomen, groin, umbilical region, LI-8, 181; KI-3, 143; ST-45, 153; LI-8, 181; BL-23, 88; ST-37, 221
pain in ankle joints, LV-4, 138; KI-2, 142
pain in area below the sternum, LV-3, 138
pain in arm and elbow, HT-5, 109; TW-3, 122; LI-13, 119; TW-1, 121; TW-10, 186
pain in arm and/or shoulder, SI-14, 186
pain in arm joints, GB-4, 224
pain in armpit and elbow, SI-8, 127
pain in arms, SI-1, 125; LU-10, 176; PC-1, 178
pain in arms, swelling and, ST-18, 46
pain in back, BL-21, 86; BL-45, 243; BL-50, 155
pain in back and loins, BL-51, 244
pain in back and spine, KI-4, 145; BL-54, 155
pain in back with chills, BL-41, 242
pain in bottom of heel, KI-7, 145
pain in chest, CV-19, 169; HT-8, 112; LU-4, 175; TW-10, 186; KI-22, 201; LI-9, 181; KI-21, 201
pain in chest and ribs, HT-1, 177
pain in chest and sides, GB-38, 163
pain in chest and stomach, SP-3, 204
pain in chest in different areas at different times, GB-43, 235
pain in chest spreading to the sides, TW-19, 189
pain in chest with chills, GB-41, 234
pain in diaphragm, SP-17, 208
pain in elbow, LI-11, 118; ST-41, 151
pain in eyebrow, BL-2, 25
pain in eyes, GB-14, 25; ST-8, 16; HT-5, 109
pain in five fingers, LU-11, 102; XFi-5, 130
pain in five fingers and weakness in hand, TW-5, 123; SI-7, 192
pain in forehead, BL-2, 25
pain in genitals, LV-3, 138
pain in groin, ST-45, 153
pain in gums, TW-2, 121; SI-8, 127
pain in heart, LV-14, 46; XT-1, 153
pain in heart area, LV-13, 48
pain in heel, KI-1, 141; KI-3, 143; ST-36, 150
pain in hip radiating to the lower abdomen, GB-25, 231
pain in inner ear, TW-21, 21
pain in inner side of arm, HT-9, 113
pain in inner thigh, LV-8, 139; KI-10, 197; SP-5, 133; KI-7, 145
pain in inner thigh/knee, SP-8, 205
pain in intestines, GV-4, 78; BL-27, 89; ST-37, 221
pain in knee, LV-8, 139; ST-35, 221; SP-3, 204; XL-1a, 149
pain in knee joint, XL-1, 148
pain in lateral side of the arms, LU-9, 101
pain in lower abdomen, BL-25, 89; KI-7, 145; ST-25, 66; BL-28, 90; KI-6, 144; SI-8, 127; SP-4, 133; GB-25, 231; LV-1, 137; LV-6, 211; LV-8, 139;
pain in lower abdomen radiating to the throat, ST-31, 220

	pain in lower abdomen/loins, BL-23, 88; ST-37, 221
	pain in lower back, GV-7, 171
	pain in neck, LU-7, 100
	pain in neck and back, BL-10, 18
	pain in neck and lower jaw, SI-8, 127
fever	pain in neck with chills and, ST-5, 214
	pain in one side of head and neck, GB-4, 224; GB-11, 227
	pain in one side of the vagina, BL-55, 245
	pain in outer side of the elbow, SI-11, 193
	pain in outer wrist, SI-4, 126
	pain in outside edge of arm, SI-5, 126
	pain in palm, LU-10, 176
	pain in penis, KI-12, 198; LU-7, 100; LV-1, 137; LV-8, 139; SP-6, 134;
	pain in ribs, BL-40, 241
	pain in scalp, ST-44, 152
	pain in shoulder and arm, TW-4, 122; TW-14, 187; LI-2, 179; BL-40, 241; GB-21, 71; LU-5, 99
	pain in shoulder and back, LU-9, 101; LI-10, 117; LU-1, 47; LU-2, 174
	pain in shoulder and elbow, SI-8, 127; LI-6, 180
back	pain in shoulder radiating to the, ST-19, 217
	pain in sides radiating to chest, SP-13, 206
	pain in small intestine, ST-30, 68
	pain in sole of foot, KI-3, 143
	pain in spine, GV-12, 76; LU-5, 99; BL-60, 158
	pain in spine and sacrum, BL-27, 89
	pain in sternum, BL-18, 85
	pain in stomach, CV-13, 52
inflammation or	pain in testicles CV-3, 61; BL-33, 92
	pain in testicles, CV-7, 57; LV-5, 211
wrist weakness or	pain in the, TW-4, 122
cutting	pain in the abdomen, ST-40, 151
	pain in the base of the skull, GB-41, 234
stabbing	pain in the chest, ST-40, 151
cannot bend	pain in the elbow, PC-3, 103
inflammation and	pain in the eyes, GB-16, 14
	pain in the five toes, LV-4, 138; KI-1, 141
knee	pain in the inner side of the, SP-6, 134
(violent)	pain in the lower abdomen, LV-5, 211
	pain in the neck and shoulder, SI-16, 194
	pain in the shoulder, LI-11, 118; BL-37, 241
	pain in the top of the head, GB-8, 226
	pain in the upper abdomen, ST-26, 219
	pain in the upper arm, LI-11, 118
like a knife turning	pain in the whole belly, CV-7, 57
	pain in the yin side of the arm, PC-6, 105
	pain in throat, LV-7, 139
	pain in upper part of the hips, GB-26, 49
	pain in uterus, GB-26, 49; KI-3, 143; ST-33, 148
	pain in vagina, CV-3, 61; ST-29, 68
	pain in wrist joint, LU-9, 101
hernia and/or	pain inflammation in testicle, CV-6, 58

	pain moving over body joints, GB-38, 163
stiffness and	pain of knuckles, XHn-1, 129
	pain of medial malleolus, LV-3, 138
	pain of penis or scrotum, LV-12, 212
	pain of skin of whole body, CV-1, 62
foreleg	pain of the inner side of the, LV-7, 139
with cold	pain of the knee, leg, and lumbago, ST-34, 220
	pain of tibia bone, KI-1, 141
feeling of oppression and	pain on the chest, LU-2, 174
cramping and	pain on the elbow, PC-7, 105
pruritis and	pain on the skin, BL-13, 83
	pain or cramp in lumbar vertebrae, CV-9, 54
	pain or inflammation in testicles, ST-27, 67
spine stiffness	pain or numbness XSP-1, 166
	pain or swelling in vagina, CV-1, 62
swelling of jaw with	pain radiating behind the ear, SI-2, 191
abdomen,	pain radiating to the lower back, GB-29, 232
low back	pain radiating to the testicles, BL-34, 92
	pain radiating to the umbilicus, ST-26, 219
ankle	pain (severe), BL-60, 158
back	pain (severe), BL-65, 249
eye	pain (severe), BL-9, 238
gastric	pain (severe), SP-5, 133
like a knife twisting	pain (sharp) in the abdomen, LI-8, 181
	pain (sharp) in the knee, KI-10, 197
scapula region	pain spreading to the, TW-13, 187
chronic chi disease gastric	pain stomachache not enough energy, CV-6, 58
	pain under the armpit, GB-42, 235
	pain under the chest (severe), BL-46, 243
blood pressure	pain under the chest with low, SP-3, 204
	pain under the heel, KI-8, 146
	pain under umbilicus, SP-6, 134
neck	pain with chills, TW-10, 186
cardiac	pain with the sensation of energy rising, CV-11, 53
abdomen	painful BL-16, 239; BL-29, 240; CV-10, 54; KI-17, 199;
head heavy and	painful, BL-59, 247
inner canthus	painful, BL-67, 159
abdomen swollen and	painful, CV-11, 53
heart and stomach	painful, CV-12, 53
chest feels hot and	painful, CV-13, 52
chest	painful, CV-14, 52; CV-18, 169; GB-10, 227; GB-43, 235;
penis feels cold and	painful, CV-1, 62
chest and ribs swollen and	painful, CV-16, 43
heart and chest	painful, CV-17, 43
breast swollen and	painful, CV-19, 169; ST-34, 220
sides of the chest full and	painful, CV-21, 170
swollen or full and extremely	painful, lower abdomenCV-2, 62
vaginal orifice swollen and	painful, CV-3, 61
lower abdomen	painful, GB-25, 231; LV-1, 137; LV-6, 211; LV-8, 139
loins and legs	painful, GB-32, 232
skin	painful, GB-36, 233
fibula	painful, GB-37, 234
lumbar and thigh	painful, GB-40, 164

cannot turn body, chest painful,, GB-43, 235
outer canthus painful, GB-44, 165
chest and sides painful, GB-44, 165; LV-2, 137
throat swollen and painful, GV-16, 17
loins and back painful, GV-9, 77; GB-27, 231
ankle joint painful, KI-6, 144
chest and back painful, LU-10, 176
loins and chest painful, PC-7, 105
neck swollen and painful, SI-10, 192; TW-12, 187
arms and shoulders sore and painful, SI-11, 193
chest full and painful, SP-18, 209; KI-24, 202
tongue stiff and painful, SP-5, 133
body feels heavy, joints painful, SP-5, 133; SP-2, 132; SP-3, 204
abdomen and sides of body painful, SP-8, 205
eyes red and painful, ST-1, 213; ST-2, 213
shoulder/ribs painful, ST-19, 217
outer corners of eyes red, painful, TW-10, 186
arms, back swollen and painful, TW-12, 187
shoulder swollen and painful, TW-13, 187
eyes red swollen and painful, TW-23, 26
skin and flesh painful, TW-7, 185
fingers numb and painful, XHn-1, 129
abdomen painful after confinement, CV-4, 60
abdomen swollen painful and hot, CV-5, 59
lower limbs painful and/or numb, SP-6, 134
heart painful as if it had been stabbed, KI-2, 142
joints painful body heavy, SP-2, 132; SP-3, 204
abdomen painful down to the sexual organs, CV-4, 60
stiff and painful finger joints, XFi-6, 130
sore and painful foot, KI-3, 143
different times leg painful in different areas, GB-41, 234
BL-23, LV-14 combined for painful intercourse, LV-14, 46
sore and painful tibia bone, LV-3, 138; ST-37, 221
chest and ribs painful cannot lie down, LV-13, 48
sore and painful shoulder and upper arm, SI-6, 191
skin too painful to wear clothes, ST-20, 218
chest painful when coughing, GB-39, 164
chest and sides full and painful with dyspnea, GB-40, 164
eyes red and painful with headache, BL-2, 25
sciatica, BL-30, 90; BL-31, 91; BL-32, 91; BL-33, 92; BL-60, 158; GB-30, 161; GB-32, 232; GB-34, 163; XL-4, 161

Point Index

Bladder Meridian

Point; Sec; Ilus; Page

BL-1; 6,4; 8; 26
BL-2; 6,2; 8; 25
BL-3; 42,1; 236
BL-4; 42,2; 236
BL-5; 42,3; 236
BL-6; 42,4; 237
BL-7; 42,5; 237
BL-8; 42,6; 238
BL-9; 42,7; 238
BL-10; 4,3; 6; 18
BL-11; 17,1; 19; 82
BL-12; 17,2; 19; 83
BL-13; 17,3; 19; 83
BL-14; 42,8; 238
BL-15; 17,4; 19; 84
BL-16; 42,9; 239
BL-17; 17,5; 19; 84
BL-18; 17,6; 19; 85
BL-19; 17,7; 19; 85
BL-20; 17,8; 19; 86
BL-21; 17,9; 19; 86
BL-22; 17,10; 19; 87
BL-23; 17,11; 19; 88
BL-24; 42,10; 239
BL-25; 17,12; 19; 89
BL-26; 42,11; 239
BL-27; 17,13; 19; 89
BL-28; 17,14; 19; 90
BL-29; 42,12; 240
BL-30; 17,15; 19; 90
BL-31; 17,16; 19; 91
BL-32; 17,17; 19; 91
BL-33; 17,18; 19; 92
BL-34; 17,19; 19; 92
BL-35; 17,20; 19; 93
BL-36; 42,13; 240
BL-37; 42,14; 241
BL-38; 18,1; 20; 95
BL-39; 42,15; 241
BL-40; 42,16; 241
BL-41; 42,17; 242
BL-42; 42,18; 242
BL-43; 42,19; 242
BL-44; 42,20; 243
BL-45; 42,21; 243
BL-46; 42,22; 243
BL-47; 18,3; 20; 97
BL-48; 42,23; 244
BL-49; 42,24; 244
BL-50; 27,1; 29; 155
BL-51; 42,25; 244
BL-52; 42,26; 245
BL-53; 42,27; 245
BL-54; 27,2; 29; 155
BL-55; 42,28; 245
BL-56; 42,29; 246
BL-57; 27,3; 29; 157
BL-58; 42,30; 246
BL-59; 42,31; 247
BL-60; 27,5; 29; 158
BL-61; 42,32; 247
BL-62; 27,6; 29; 158
BL-63; 27,7; 29; 159
BL-64; 42,33; 248
BL-65; 42,34; 249
BL-66; 42,35; 249
BL-67; 27,8; 29; 159

Conception Vessel Meridian

Point; Sec; Ilus; Page

CV-1; 13,7; 15; 62
CV-2; 13,6; 15; 62
CV-3; 13,5; 15; 61
CV-4; 13,4; 15; 60
CV-5; 13,3; 15; 59
CV-6; 13,2; 15; 58
CV-7; 13,1; 15; 57
CV-8; 12,8; 14; 55
CV-9; 12,7; 14; 54
CV-10; 12,6; 14; 54
CV-11; 12,5; 14; 53
CV-12; 12,4; 14; 53
CV-13; 12,3; 14; 52
CV-14; 12,2; 14; 52
CV-15; 12,1; 14; 51
CV-16; 10,4; 12; 43
CV-17; 10,3; 12; 43
CV-18; 29,1; 169
CV-19; 29,2; 169
CV-20; 29,3; 170

CV-21; 29,4; 170
CV-22; 10,2; 12; 42
CV-23; 10,1; 12; 41
CV-24; 8,3; 10; 32

Gallbladder Meridian

Point; Sec; Ilus; Page
GB-1; 6,5; 8; 27
GB-2; 5,2; 7; 21
GB-3; 41,1; 224
GB-4; 41,2; 224
GB-5; 41,3; 225
GB-6; 41,4; 225
GB-7; 41,5; 226
GB-8; 41,6; 226
GB-9; 41,7; 226
GB-10; 41,8; 227
GB-11; 41,9; 227
GB-12; 41,10; 228
GB-13; 3,1; 6; 16
GB-14; 6,1; 8; 25
GB-15; 2,1; 5; 14
GB-16; 2,2; 5; 14
GB-17; 41,11; 228
GB-18; 41,12; 228
GB-19; 41,13; 229
GB-20; 4,4; 6; 19
GB-21; 15,1; 17; 71
GB-22; 41,14; 229
GB-23; 41,15; 230
GB-24; 41,16; 230
GB-25; 41,17; 231
GB-26; 11,7; 13; 49
GB-27; 41,18; 231
GB-28; 41,19; 232
GB-29; 41,20; 232
GB-30; 28,1; 30; 161
GB-31; 28,3; 30; 162
GB-32; 41,21; 232
GB-33; 28,4; 30; 162
GB-34; 28,5; 30; 163
GB-35; 41,22; 233
GB-36; 41,23; 233
GB-37; 41,24; 234
GB-38; 28,6; 30; 163
GB-39; 28,7; 30; 164
GB-40; 28,8; 30; 164
GB-41; 41,25; 234
GB-42; 41,26; 235
GB-43; 41,27; 235
GB-44; 28,9; 30; 165

Governing Vessel Meridian

Point; Sec; Ilus; Page
GV-1; 16,10; 18; 80
GV-2; 16,9; 18; 79
GV-3; 16,8; 18; 79
GV-4; 16,7; 18; 78
GV-5; 30,1; 171
GV-6; 30,2; 171
GV-7; 30,3; 171
GV-8; 30,4; 172
GV-9; 16,6; 18; 77
GV-10; 16,5; 18; 77
GV-11; 16,4; 18; 76
GV-12; 16,3; 18; 76
GV-13; 16,2; 18; 75
GV-14; 16,1; 18; 74
GV-15; 4,2; 6; 18
GV-16; 4,1; 6; 17
GV-17; 30,5; 172
GV-18; 30,6; 172
GV-19; 1,6; 5; 13
GV-20; 1,5; 5; 13
GV-21; 1,4; 5; 12
GV-22; 1,3; 5; 12
GV-23; 1,2; 5; 11
GV-24; 1,1; 5; 11
GV-25; 7,1; 9; 29
GV-26; 8,1; 10; 31
GV-27; 30,7; 173
GV-28; 30,8; 173

Heart Meridian

Point; Sec; Ilus; Page
HT-1; 32,1; 177
HT-2; 32,2; 177
HT-3; 19,14; 21; 108
HT-4; 19,15; 21; 109
HT-5; 19,16; 21; 109
HT-6; 19,17; 21; 110
HT-7; 19,18; 21; 111
HT-8; 19,19; 21; 112
HT-9; 19,20; 21; 113

Kidney Meridian

Point; Sec; Ilus; Page

KI-1; 25,1; 27; 141
KI-2; 25,2; 27; 142
KI-3; 25,3; 27; 143
KI-4; 25,5; 27; 145
KI-5; 37,1; 196
KI-6; 25,4; 27; 144
KI-7; 25,6; 27; 145
KI-8; 25,7; 27; 146
KI-9; 37,2; 196
KI-10; 37,3; 197
KI-11; 37,4; 197
KI-12; 37,5; 198
KI-13; 37,6; 198
KI-14; 37,7; 198
KI-15; 37,8; 199
KI-16; 37,9; 199
KI-17; 37,10; 199
KI-18; 37,11; 200
KI-19; 37,12; 200
KI-20; 37,13; 200
KI-21; 37,14; 201
KI-22; 37,15; 201
KI-23; 37,16; 201
KI-24; 37,17; 202
KI-25; 37,18; 202
KI-26; 37,19; 202
KI-27; 37,20; 203

Large Intestine Meridian

Point; Sec; Ilus; Page

LI-1; 20,1; 22; 115
LI-2; 34,1; 179
LI-3; 34,2; 179
LI-4; 20,2; 22; 115
LI-5; 20,3; 22; 116
LI-6; 34,3; 180
LI-7; 34,4; 180
LI-8; 34,5; 181
LI-9; 34,6; 181
LI-10; 20,4; 22; 117
LI-11; 20,5; 22; 118
LI-12; 34,7; 182
LI-13; 20,6; 22; 119
LI-14; 20,7; 22; 119
LI-15; 15,2; 17; 72
LI-16; 15,3; 17; 72
LI-17; 34,8; 183
LI-18; 34,9; 183
LI-19; 34,10; 184
LI-20; 7,2; 9; 29

Lung Meridian

Point; Sec; Ilus; Page

LU-1; 11,5; 13; 47
LU-2; 31,1; 174
LU-3; 31,2; 174
LU-4; 31,3; 175
LU-5; 19,1; 21; 99
LU-6; 31,4; 175
LU-7; 19,2; 21; 100
LU-8; 19,3; 21; 101
LU-9; 19,4; 21; 101
LU-10; 31,5; 176
LU-11; 19,5; 21; 102

Liver Meridian

Point; Sec; Ilus; Page

LV-1; 24,1; 26; 137
LV-2; 24,2; 26; 137
LV-3; 24,3; 26; 138
LV-4; 24,4; 26; 138
LV-5; 39,1; 211
LV-6; 39,2; 211
LV-7; 24,5; 26; 139
LV-8; 24,6; 26; 139
LV-9; 39,3; 212
LV-10; 39,4; 212
LV-11; 14,6; 16; 69
LV-12; 39,5; 212
LV-13; 11,6; 13; 48
LV-14; 11,4; 13; 46

Pericardium Meridian

Point; Sec; Ilus; Page

PC-1; 33,1; 178
PC-2; 33,2; 178
PC-3; 19,6; 21; 103
PC-4; 19,7; 21; 103
PC-5; 19,9; 21; 104
PC-6; 19,10; 21; 105
PC-7; 19,11; 21; 105
PC-8; 21; 106;
PC-9; 19,13; 21; 107

Small Intestine Meridian

Point; Sec; Ilus; Page

SI-1; 22,1; 24; 125
SI-2; 36,1; 191
SI-3; 22,2; 24; 125
SI-4; 22,3; 24; 126
SI-5; 22,4; 24; 126
SI-6; 36,2; 191
SI-7; 36,3; 192
SI-8; 22,5; 24; 127
SI-9; 36,4; 192
SI-10; 36,5; 192
SI-11; 36,6; 193
SI-12; 36,7; 193
SI-13; 36,8; 193
SI-14; 36,9; 194
SI-15; 36,10; 194
SI-16; 36,11; 194
SI-17; 36,12; 195
SI-18; 36,13; 195
SI-19; 5,3; 7; 22

Spleen Meridian

Point; Sec; Ilus; Page

SP-1; 23,1; 25; 132
SP-2; 23,2; 25; 132
SP-3; 38,1; 204
SP-4; 23,3; 25; 133
SP-5; 23,4; 25; 133
SP-6; 23,5; 25; 134
SP-7; 38,2; 204
SP-8; 38,3; 205
SP-9; 23,6; 25; 135
SP-10; 23,7; 25; 135
SP-11; 38,4; 205
SP-12; 38,5; 206
SP-13; 38,6; 206
SP-14; 38,7; 207
SP-15; 38,8; 207
SP-16; 38,9; 208
SP-17; 38,10; 208
SP-18; 38,11; 209
SP-19; 38,12; 209
SP-20; 38,13; 210
SP-21; 38,14; 210

Stomach Meridian

Point; Sec; Ilus; Page

ST-1; 40,1; 213
ST-2; 40,2; 213
ST-3; 40,3; 214
ST-4; 8,2; 10; 31
ST-5; 40,4; 214
ST-6; 5,5; 7; 23
ST-7; 40,5; 215
ST-8; 3,2; 6; 16
ST-9; 40,6; 215
ST-10; 40,7; 216
ST-11; 40,8; 216
ST-12; 11,1; 13; 45
ST-13; 40,9; 216
ST-14; 40,10; 217
ST-15; 40,11; 217
ST-16; 11,2; 13; 45
ST-18; 11,3; 13; 46
ST-19; 40,12; 217
ST-20; 40,13; 218
ST-21; 40,14; 218
ST-22; 40,15; 218
ST-23; 40,16; 219
ST-24; 40,17; 219
ST-25; 14,1; 16; 66
ST-26; 40,18; 219
ST-27; 14,2; 16; 67
ST-28; 14,3; 16; 67
ST-29; 14,4; 16; 68
ST-30; 14,5; 16; 68
ST-31; 40,19; 220
ST-32; 40,20; 220
ST-33; 26,1; 28; 148
ST-34; 40,21; 220
ST-35; 40,22; 221
ST-36a; 26,6; 28; 150
ST-36; 26,5; 28; 150
ST-37; 40,23; 221
ST-38; 40,24; 222
ST-39; 40,25; 222
ST-40; 26,7; 28; 151
ST-41; 26,8; 28; 151
ST-42; 26,9; 28; 152
ST-43; 40,26; 223
ST-44; 26,10; 28; 152
ST-45; 26,11; 28; 153

Triple Warmer Meridian

Point; Sec; Ilus; Page

TW-1; 21,1; 23; 121
TW-2; 21,2; 23; 121
TW-3; 21,3; 23; 122
TW-4; 21,4; 23; 122
TW-5; 21,5; 23; 123
TW-6; 21,6; 23; 123
TW-7; 35,1; 185
TW-8; 35,2; 185
TW-9; 35,3; 185
TW-10; 35,4; 186
TW-11; 35-5; 186
TW-12; 35,6; 187
TW-13; 35,7; 187
TW-14; 35,8; 187
TW-15; 35,9; 188
TW-16; 35,10; 188
TW-17; 5,4; 7; 22
TW-18; 35,11; 189
TW-19; 35,12; 189
TW-20; 35,13; 190
TW-21; 5,1; 7; 21
TW-22; 35,14; 190
TW-23; 6,3; 8; 26

Extra Points

Point; Sec; Ilus; Page

XA-1; 19,8; 21; 104
XA-2; 22,6; 24; 127
XB-1; 18,2; 20; 96
XB-2; 18,4; 20; 97
XF-1; 9,6; 11; 36
XF-2; 9,7; 11; 37
XF-3; 9,8; 11; 37
XF-4; 9,9; 11; 38
XF-5; 9,10; 11; 38
XF-6; 9,11; 11; 38
XF-7; 9,12; 11; 39
XF-8 (l.); 9,13; 11; 39
XF-8 (r.); 9,14; 11; 39
XFi-1; 19,21; 21; 113
XFi-2; 22,7; 24; 128
XFi-3; 22,8; 24; 128
XFi-4; 22,10; 24; 129
XFi-5; 22,11; 24; 130
XFi-6; 22,12; 24; 130
XFo-1; 28,10; 30; 165
XH-1; 9,2; 11; 34
XH-2; 9,3; 11; 35
XH-3; 9,4; 11; 35
XH-4; 9,5; 11; 36
XHn-1; 22,9; 24; 129
XL-1a; 26,3; 28; 149
XL-1; 26,2; 28; 148
XL-2; 26,4; 28; 149
XL-3; 27,4; 29; 157
XL-4; 28,2; 30; 161
XN-1; 9,1; 11; 34
XP-1; 13,9; 15; 64
XSC-1; 13,8; 15; 63
XSP-1; 28,11; 30; 166
XT-1; 26,12; 28; 153